RESUSCITATING U.S. HEALTHCARE

An Insider's Manifesto for Reform

Steve Parker, M.D.

pxHealth

First edition published 2024
ISBN: 9780989477543

Published by pxHealth
29455 N. Cave Creek Road
Suite 118-288
Cave Creek, AZ 85331 USA

Dedicated to
Brian Puente and Sunny Parker,
who learned way too much about U.S.
healthcare., the hard way

CONTENTS

PREFACE

The current U.S. healthcare system is cruel, abusive, insulting, and corrupt. It must change. It will change. But will changes be to the benefit of healthcare consumers or to the profiteers?

U.S. healthcare spending in 2022 was $4.5 trillion, or ~$13,500 per person. Seventeen percent of U.S. Gross Domestic Product goes to healthcare. That's almost one in every six dollars. We are not that sick, people! Too many of those dollars are providing obscene profit or wasted on administrative costs that don't benefit patients.

As a full-time practicing physician (internist) for over forty years, I've observed this "system" up close and personal. "Non-system" would be more accurate. Like my patients, I've been a pawn in a 3-D chess game, often not knowing who's moving the chess pieces.

U.S. healthcare is cruel. Examples?

- Hospitals kicking patients out too soon.
- Patients denied the most effective medication because "it's not on the formulary" of their insurance plan or it's prohibitively expensive.
- Denial of insurance coverage for a cutting-edge (and better) procedure because it's more expensive than the old ways.
- Physicians providing poor care, not because of ignorance, but because providing good care is time-consuming and the doctor gets paid more for simply seeing more patients, too many patients.
- Mental health providers and primary care physicians just prescribe more and more drugs when talk therapy would be more effective.
- Patients denied necessary ongoing physical therapy because they reached their insurance limit.
- Patients sued into bankruptcy by wealthy healthcare providers, even non-profit corporations, when everybody knows the patient has no way to ever pay their bills.

U.S. healthcare is abusive. Examples?

- Endless time on telephone or online "hold" when the consumer needs answers to even simple questions.
- Healthcare providers and insurers deliberately using pretentious jargon to confuse consumers.
- Insurers refusing to pay for necessary services

until multiple less expensive options have been tried and failed, while the patient suffers.

- Patients being forced to change healthcare providers away from those they've known and trusted for years.

- Healthcare organizations or insurers offering panels of providers not because they're the best, but the cheapest.

- Providers not being able to state the price of care before it's rendered, not even a ballpark estimate.

- Providers not explaining the pros and cons of a particular therapeutic course of action, nor the alternatives.

- Politicians requiring consumers to pay for insurance coverage that they don't want and will never use.

- Politicians and insurers setting provider pay rates so low that, even though they have "coverage," the patient can't find a provider willing to see them.

- Excessively long wait times for an appointment while the suffering is ongoing.

- Deliberate over-complexity of a system so the consumer can't figure out what's going on (while getting sheared like a sheep).

U.S. healthcare is insulting. Examples?

- Delay in care by forcing a patient to see a primary care provider when the patient (and even the PCP) knows damn well she needs a specialist.

- Patients being treated like cattle, with a number not a name, a "case" rather than a fellow human deserving dignity.

- Insurers and healthcare organizations assuming patients can't figure out who are the good providers in their community and who's in the bottom 20%.

- Politicians, providers, and insurers treating consumers as if they were children.

- Politicians, insurers, and bureaucrats interfering with the patient-physician relationship as if they know what's best for the patient.

- Employers choosing health plans with little or no input from the workers.

U.S. healthcare is corrupt. Examples?

- Healthcare organizations and insurers spending billions of dollars to influence legislation to their own benefit, not the consumer's.

- Politicians taking bribes and campaign contributions in order to screw the consumer, who doesn't have a lobbyist or much money.

- Bureaucrats and politicians neglecting care of our veterans for years until the evidence is just too overwhelming to ignore.

- Judges changing the clear meaning of written words in order to favor corporations over the little guy.

- Expert witnesses for malpractice lawsuits lying under oath simply for a hefty paycheck.

- Pharmaceutical companies lying about the addiction potential of opioids, in service of pure profit.

WHAT IS A HEALTHCARE PROVIDER?

If you are easily bored and already know what a healthcare provider is, skip this paragraph. But for clarity's sake: Healthcare providers include physicians, physician assistants, nurse practitioners, hospitals and other healthcare systems (HMOs, PPOs, ACOs, etc), freestanding emergency departments, urgent care centers, pharmacists and pharmacies, medical labs and diagnostic facilities, medical imaging facilities, physical therapists and their companies, speech therapists and their companies, occupational therapists and their companies, DME (durable medical equipment) suppliers, hospices, psychologists, psychiatric social workers, nursing homes, skilled nursing facilities, long-term acute care facilities, ambulances/EMTs/paramedics, patient transporters (overland or in the air), and fire departments that make medical calls, for example.

We can't ignore health insurers in this discussion. Pure insurers are not healthcare providers. But some healthcare delivery systems function as both insurers and healthcare providers. The other major players in the U.S. healthcare non-system are pharmaceutical companies, politicians, and bureaucrats. The latter may work for private companies or the government.

In its purest form, healthcare is a patient-physician relationship. Generally, a patient comes to me with an ailment. I do an assessment, establish a diagnosis, and recommend a course of action. The patient can accept or reject my recommendations, which may involve other healthcare providers. As an internist, I don't do surgery or many other procedures. My recommendations to the patient, for example, may involve medications, lifestyle changes, hospitalization, physical therapy, diagnostic testing in a lab or imaging facility, or referral to another physician for a procedure or second opinion. These other folks that I get involved in this patient-physician relationship are all healthcare providers. Physicians aren't the only providers.

Rather than seeing a physician from the get-go, the patient may opt instead to see a nurse practitioner, physician assistant, physical therapist, psychologist, massage therapist, nutritionist, chiropractor, hypnotist, acupuncturist, naturopath, aroma therapist, exorcist, shaman, or a number of other practitioners or providers. Some of these non-physician healthcare providers and their treatments undoubtedly will be beneficial or curative to the patient. So I'm willing to expand the concept of "patient-physician relationship" to "patient-provider relationship."

I'm also willing to admit that a patient is a consumer, even a customer, of healthcare.

Going forward, for purposes of this manifesto, I'm restricting the term "healthcare providers" to only those whose services are science-based. Due to their training and experience, MD and DO physicians are the logical ones to decide, by consensus, which tests and treatments are science-based. Yes, the science changes over time as new data become available; that's the nature of science. Health insurance should only pay for science-based evaluation and care.

I considered defining healthcare for you but that's too pedantic. Like pornography, most people know it when they see it. In my example of the patient-physician relationship, I referred to a patient having an ailment. To be sure, healthcare also includes health maintenance and preventative care.

WHY CALL A "CODE BLUE" AND RESUSCITATE U.S. HEALTHCARE NOW?

Despite consumers putting up with cruelty, abuse, insults, and corruption, the U.S. healthcare system is by far the most costly in the world. Comparing our health outcomes to the rest of the world, the results don't justify the cost.

And we can't afford it any longer.

Almost one in every six dollars is spent on healthcare. We have an aging population that will need more healthcare than when they were younger. Federal spending is spiraling out of control and a large chunk of that is for healthcare. States' budgets would be just as unbalanced if only they could print money. Deficit spending will cripple the economy, either for us or our children.

Again, if we were a sickly people, we'd gladly spend lots on healthcare if it would make us feel better and live longer. But we're not getting the expected return on investment.

By the way, I'm about to use my first Reference. References are numbers in parentheses and are listed near the end of this book under, you guessed it, "References."

A Gallup survey (9) in 2021 found that 100 million U.S. adults described the healthcare system as "expensive" or "broken." Nearly a third of surveyed adults reported that they skipped needed healthcare due to cost. 42% were concerned that they wouldn't be able to pay for healthcare in the coming year. Over half said that the cost of healthcare contributed some (36%) or a lot (15%) of stress to their daily lives. Nearly one half reported that the COVID-19 pandemic worsened their view of healthcare.

Despite spending more money per capita than any other wealthy country, **Americans don't grade their system overall very highly in terms of A through F.** According to a 2023 Harris Poll survey (76), "More than half of the roughly 2,500 U.S. adults who took the survey graded the U.S. health care system a "C" or below. When asked about factors that prevent people in the U.S. from getting care, cost was the most common criticism, followed by the system's focus on profits, inaccessibility of insurance coverage, and confusion around what is covered by insurance." Other issues were lack of timely appointments, limitations on insurance coverage, and inadequate focus on prevention and wellness.

The public doesn't seem to be tuned in to the excessive complexity of healthcare delivery. That's because most of it is handled out of sight by healthcare providers, insurance companies, and government insurance programs (e.g., Medicare and Medicaid). But consumers are definitely paying for that complexity via administrative costs passed on through high prices, premiums, and/or taxes.

The largest healthcare cost for folks who aren't very sick is actually *health insurance*. For instance, a physician friend of mine works for an employer who partially pays for a high-deductible PPO health insurance for his family (him and his wife and two dependents). My friend trusts his employer did their due diligence while shopping for the insurance, juggling price, coverage, and quality. The employer pays for my friend's personal insurance premium but the premiums for the other three are deducted from his pay. The premium for his wife and two kids is $1,204/month or $14,448 per year. Remember, that's the premium for just three people. As long as they use in-network providers, the deductible per person is $500/year and per family is $1,000/year. Their out-of-pocket limit is $11,000/year. If they choose out-of-network providers, the deductible per person escalates to $5,000 and per family to $10,000. My friend tells me he and his family are blessed with good health and they rarely use their insurance. If insurance weren't so expensive, my friend would have a higher paycheck to use as he sees fit.

Can you think of better things to spend your money on than enriching huge corporations, bureaucrats, and plutocrats?

Whether by design or haphazard, our current healthcare system is unsustainably complicated, riddled with perverse incentives, and strangled by third-party interference with the patient-provider relationship. Let's fix it.

IS THE SYSTEM ROTTEN TO THE CORE?

Absolutely not.

Healthcare undoubtedly prolongs lives, saves lives, and

alleviates suffering.

All the involved players have done good. I've seen innumerable front-line healthcare workers – nurses, respiratory therapists, patient care technicians, physicians, paramedics and EMTs (emergency medical technicians) – jeopardize their own health and lives to help others without thought of personal gain. I've seen hospital administrators in endless meetings, planning how to best protect their communities in the face of unprecedented epidemics, losing sleep at night out of worry. I've seen pharmaceutical companies produce incredible life-saving drugs that cost millions to bring to market. I've seen pharmacists make calls to prescribing physicians about life-threatening drug interactions and contra-indications that the doc missed. I've seen committees struggle for hours, days, and weeks over quality improvement initiatives. I've seen hospitals and physicians write-off huge unpayable debts from patients. I've seen physicians take out loans so they could pay their staff, while Medicare mysteriously delayed payment for months. I've seen bureaucrats and clerks go well beyond the call of duty to ensure that a patient got what they needed and deserved despite obstacles. I've seen politicians make healthcare available to suffering patients who had no other options. I'll even admit that trial lawyers have helped physicians and hospitals improve their care!

I'm proud and fortunate to have been a part of this wacky system for so many years.

But we can and should do better.

CHAPTER 1: SCOPE OF THE PROBLEM

The U.S. is easily #1 in healthcare spending compared to other modern high-income countries. But we're not getting our money's worth. In 2022, the U.S. devoted 17.3% of its gross domestic product to healthcare (59, 61, & 75), compared to 9% in 1980 and just 5% in 1960. The 17.3% is down a bit from the prior year. Here are the percentages of GDP spent on healthcare over decades:

- 1960: 5%
- 1970: 6.9%
- 1980: 8.9%
- 1990: 12.1%
- 2000: 13.3%

- 2010: 17.4%
- 2020: 18%

Despite those expenditures for healthcare, a 2023 Investopedia article (1) mentions that average life expectancy at birth in the U.S is 76.4 years. It's been falling for the last couple years and is quite a bit lower than most other high-income countries such as 80.4 years in the U.K. and 85.4 in Japan (77). Furthermore, the Centers for Disease Control reported in 2023 that infant mortality in the U.S. rose for the first time in 20 years (101). The Investopedia article also notes that only 91.4% of the population in the U.S. has health insurance, compared to 99% to 100% of the population in the other high-income countries.

A 2021 report by The Commonwealth Fund (2) compared performance of the healthcare systems in Australia, Canada, France, Germany, the Netherlands, New Zealand, Norway, Sweden, Switzerland, the United Kingdom, and the United States. Directly from the abstract:

- **Methods:** Analysis of 71 performance measures across five domains — access to care, care process, administrative efficiency, equity, and health care outcomes — drawn from Commonwealth Fund international surveys conducted in each country and administrative data from the Organisation for Economic Co-operation and Development and the World Health Organization.

- **Key Findings:** The top-performing countries overall are Norway, the Netherlands, and Australia. The United States ranks last overall, despite spending far more of its gross domestic product on health care. The U.S. ranks last on access to care, administrative efficiency, equity, and health care outcomes, but ranks second on measures of care process.

For what it's worth, the World Health Organization in way back in 2000 published their Overall Efficiency rankings for healthcare in 191 countries (6). France was #1. Sandwiched between Costa Rica and Slovenia, the U.S. was #37. We were below the 10 other high-income countries in the Commonwealth Fund study except for #41 New Zealand.

An article at BMC Health Services Research (52) mentioned that this WHO study:

…has been criticized for its objectives, confounding of social influences with health care system performance, poor data quality, and narrow scope in methodology. Some of these critics re-estimated efficiency and rankings, using different approaches, which generally led to different rankings. The US tended to rank higher in these newer studies, although none placed the US at the top.

In 2023, *U.S. News and World Report* published a list (7) of "the most well-developed public health systems" based on a survey of 17,000 global citizens. Belgium earned the #1 spot. Most of the 10 other high-income countries in the The Commonwealth Fund study were in the Top 10 of this ranking. The U.S. came in at #23, between Italy and Portugal.

The Legatum Prosperity Index (100) is about "advancing the understanding of what drives success in [167] nations." The index has 12 pillars, including health, which "measures the extent to which people are healthy and have access to the necessary services to maintain good health, including health outcomes, health systems, illness and risk factors, and mortality rates." So a country's healthcare system is only one contributor to health. Other related factors would include genetics, geography, environmental pollution, political system, etc. For what it's worth, in 2023 the Index's Health Pillar ranked Singapore #1, Japan #2, South Korea #3, Taiwan #4, Norway #7, Sweden #9, Switzerland #10, Netherlands #11, Germany #13, Hong Kong #14, Italy #17, France #20, Australia #21, New Zealand #25, Canada #32, U.K. #34, Malaysia #42, United States #69.

USA! USA! We're #1! We're #1! Well, we're #1 in cost for sure. But quality?

A 2020 report from The Commonwealth Fund (5) looked at limited health data from the Organisation for Economic Co-operation and Development (OECD) to assess the U.S. healthcare system relative to 10 other high-income countries: Australia, Canada, France, Germany, the Netherlands, New Zealand, Norway, Sweden, Switzerland, and the United Kingdom. They also compared U.S. performance to that of the OECD average, comprising 36 high-income member countries.

- While spending almost twice as much as the average OECD country, the U.S. had the lowest life expectancy and highest suicide rate among the 11 nations
- The U.S. had an obesity rate that is twice the OECD average, and the highest overall chronic

disease burden
- U.S. residents had fewer physician visits than those in most countries
- U.S. residents use some expensive technologies, such as MRIs, and specialized procedures, such as hip replacements, more often than our peers
- Compared to the other 10 OECD nations, the U.S. had among the highest number of hospitalizations from preventable causes and the highest rate of avoidable deaths

So of these 11 high-income countries, the U.S. ranks #1 in lowest life expectancy, suicides, overall chronic disease burden, and highest avoidable deaths. But wait, there's more! We're also #1 in corruption, according to Transparency International's Corruption Perception Index (116).

CHAPTER 2:
CAUSES OF HIGH HEALTHCARE AND HEALTH INSURANCE COSTS

First let's look at where the money - $4,500,000,000,000 ($4.5 trillion) in 2022 - is going or coming from (59). By the way, that $4.5 trillion is $13,500 per person, which is about twice as much as the average high-income country. Yet we score poorly on longevity, suicides, maternal mortality, and preventable hospital admissions. Astoundingly, the U.S.

accounts for 40% of global healthcare spending (80).

What were the sources of that $4.5 trillion national health expenditure? By percentage:

- Private health insurance 29%
- Medicare 21%
- Medicaid 18%
- Other 3rd party payers and programs and public health activity 13%
- Out of pocket spending 11%

(The total is over 100% due to category overlap)

Who are the major payers of healthcare costs by percentage?

- Federal government 33%
- Households 28%
- Private business share 18%
- State and local government 15%
- Other private revenues 7%

To effectively cure or treat a disease, it's immensely helpful if the physician has an accurate diagnosis. Knowing the diagnosis often tells us the underlying disease mechanism, which we can attack with specific medications, surgery, nutrition, physical therapy, etc. So if we want to reduce the high cost of U.S. healthcare, let's diagnose the underlying causes. What are the causes? Depends on who you ask....

For example, Harvard faculty member David Cutler (78) blames:

- High administrative costs (a third of total

healthcare expenditures, which is twice that of other high-income countries)
- Greed and gouging
- Higher utilization of healthcare resources (not that Americans seek care more often than others, but when they enter the system, intensity of care is ramped up)

Causes listed in an article by Maura Hohman in *Today* (79):

- The "for-profit insurance system," which is not at all common in other high-income countries
- Lack of guaranteed universal healthcare coverage
- Care is highly fragmented, leading to high administrative costs
- "Pay per service" which encourages over-utilization (an example of perverse incentive)
- Lack of government regulation
- Consolidation of insurance and hospital systems, which reduces competition

A *Harvard Gazette* (81) article lists key drivers of U.S. healthcare spending compared to other high-income countries:

- Administrative complexity (planning, regulating, managing health systems and services)
- Much higher cost of drugs
- High physician salaries (general practitioners, for example)

An *Investopedia* (1) article attributes high cost to:

- Multiple systems, leading to high complexity
- High drug prices compared to other countries
- High salaries for medical professionals, including nurses, compared to other high-income countries
- Profit-driven hospitals (hospitals account for 31% of national health expenditures)
- Defensive medical practices (e.g., unnecessary tests and scans)
- Varying healthcare prices

The Peter G. Peterson Foundation (82) posits that high cost is due to:

- An aging population that naturally requires more healthcare
- Increasing prices of healthcare services, perhaps due to 1) new, innovative technology, 2) complexity leading to administrative waste, and 3) consolidation of hospitals leading to reduced competition.

A Commonwealth Fund article (83) compared U.S. healthcare spending to peer nations, looking for the explanation for the excess cost of the U.S. system.

They explain over 50% of it with:

- U.S. pays more in administrative costs of insurance (15% share of excess spending)
- U.S. healthcare providers spend more time on administrative activities (15% share)
- U.S. pays more for prescription drugs (10% share)
- U.S. physicians earn more (10% share)

- U.S. nurses earn more (5% share)
- U.S. invests more in medical machinery and equipment (5% share)

The Research and Action Institute of AAMC (Association of American Medical Colleges) published a position paper (84) identifying high cost due to:

- Prices charged for services are too high
- Wages of clinicians are too high

Dr. Peter Ubel in an article at *Forbes* (85) argues that high healthcare cost is mainly due to:

- Lobbying by the American Medical Association, the American Hospital association, PhMRA (the primary pharmaceutical lobbying organization)

Is the cost of healthcare higher in the U.S. because we simply use healthcare services more? No, according to an article in *JAMA Network* in 2018 (3):

The United States spent approximately twice as much as other high-income countries on medical care, yet utilization rates in the United States were largely similar to those in other nations.

A 2018 article at CNBC.com (4) has additional details on the *JAMA Network* article above:

The U.S. is famous for over-spending on health care. The nation spent 17.8 percent of its GDP on health care in 2016. Meanwhile, the average spending of 11 high-income countries assessed in a new report published in the *Journal of the American Medical Association* — Canada, Germany, Australia, the U.K,. Japan, Sweden,

France, the Netherlands, Switzerland, Denmark and the U.S. — was only 11.5 percent.

Per capita, the U.S. spent $9,403. That's nearly double what the others spent.

This finding offers a new explanation as to why America's spending is so excessive. According to the researchers at the Harvard Chan School, what sets the U.S. apart may be inflated prices across the board.

In the U.S., they point out, drugs are more expensive. Doctors get paid more. Hospital services and diagnostic tests cost more. And a lot more money goes to planning, regulating and managing medical services at the administrative level.

A *Yale Insights* article (8) from 2016 focused on cost of care provided by hospitals to patients that had private insurance. So when you read "healthcare provider(s)" below, think "hospitals." Quoting Yale Professor Zack Cooper:

> This study tells us that insurance premiums are so high because healthcare provider prices are incredibly high. The way to rein in the cost of healthcare services is by targeting the massive variation in providers' prices. We can do that by making prices more transparent, making these markets more dynamic, and really blunting the monopoly power that a lot of large healthcare providers have, which has allowed them to raise prices.

Professor Cooper says the hospital industry is 8% of GDP (gross domestic product).

Let's take a deeper dive into these issues and more. You'll

notice that certain issues fall under multiple categories of cost escalation. For instance, government meddling could be categorized as "third-party interference" or "high administrative costs."

By the way, I tend to reject all explanations of high-cost care that simply say "because the prices are higher." That's like saying a Michelin 3-star restaurant is more expensive than Taco Bell because they charge higher prices. There are very good reasons the 3-star restaurant must and can charge higher prices than Taco Bell.

We need to go beyond simply saying that U.S. healthcare is more expensive because "the prices are higher" and ask *why* the prices are higher.

1. LACK OF PRICE TRANSPARENCY

Imagine going into a restaurant for a meal and there are no prices on the menu. You ask the waiter about that and he says, "Don't worry about it. We'll figure it out after you eat." You ask for a ballpark figure for the spaghetti, roasted brussels sprouts, garlic bread, and tira misu. He answers, "I don't really know. It's up to the chef and he's busy now. Don't worry, we'll take care of you." Then you get your food, it's OK, probably not something you'd order again, though. Time to settle up. "Will you be paying by cash, VISA, Mastercard, or American Express?" The waiter takes your card and, after an hour, returns with the check. You're shocked at the $254.27 price. Later you find out that the tab depends on which of those payment methods you used, and ranged from $11.50 to $2,814.05. Paying for healthcare in the U.S. is like that. Look at the bright side: at least you don't pay sales tax on healthcare!

Imagine you're driving your Corolla after dropping the kids off at school and notice you're getting dangerously low on gas. But none of the gas stations you pass have the price posted. You pull into a station to gas up, but first ask a clerk "How much is the regular gas?" Chewing gum loudly and not looking up from the register, "I dunno. It'll be on your credit card statement." Desperate to not run out of gas, you fill 'er up. A month later, you nearly faint when you get your credit card statement. Paying for healthcare in the U.S. is like that.

Imagine you're 62-years-old and that right knee soccer injury from your college days has turned into a bad case of chronic arthritis. It hurts all the time and isn't responding much to conservative therapy. Your mobility is impaired but not enough to get you "on disability," so your life sucks. Your orthopedist, whom you love and trust, says it's time for knee replacement surgery. Unfortunately, you don't have health insurance. But you do have savings. Your orthopedist is on staff at two hospitals and an outpatient surgery center. You google-search "cost of knee replacement surgery" and come up with a range of $30,000 to $60,000! You call all three facilities where your surgeon works and try to get their price for the knee surgery. You get the same old run-around: "It depends. It's hard to say. Depends on how many days in the hospital, how much physical therapy you get, the anesthesiologist's fee, the radiologist's fee, operating room fee, how much blood work, how much Tylenol and other drugs you take, any complications that arise...," etc. If you're very lucky, you'll get a range of potential total cost, but not often in writing. You only have $20,000 in savings and decide to "just tough it out" until you're on Medicare. By then, you figure you'll need an opioid addiction program, too! Paying for healthcare in the U.S. is like that. (The Surgery Center of Oklahoma is bucking the system. On January 26, 2024, I checked their online cash price for knee replacement surgery: $18,119, seemingly all-inclusive.)

Imagine you have a sore throat, fever of 101, and a cough. You need to see your primary care physician (PCP) or go to an urgent care center. It's early in the year, you haven't gotten any medical care this year, and you have a $3,000 deductible on your health insurance. This means your insurance isn't going to pay anything until you pay the first $3,000 of the year. You figure you just need a quick office visit and a strep test. Being on a budget and knowing healthcare can be expensive, you call your PCP office to ask how much this might cost. After 20 minutes on hold, the clerk is going to tell you, "I don't know for sure. It depends." Some of the "it depends" are: 1) do you have health insurance, 2) what kind of insurance, 3) the doctor may want a chest x-ray or blood work, and 4) are you paying cash and leaving insurance out of the equation. Call the Urgent Care center and you'll get the same answer about cost. When you tell either facility your insurance info, there's a fair chance they'll say, "We don't take that insurance." If you decide to just go to the hospital emergency department instead, your bill is now 10 times higher. Hey, at least you'll reach your deductible! Paying for healthcare in the U.S. is like that.

Imagine if you could go online and look up prices for a 15-minute office visit, strep throat test, and chest x-ray at the PCP's office, urgent care center, and emergency department. Online reviews and word-of-mouth are good for all three facilities. You decide where to go based on the posted prices. Paying for healthcare in the U.S. is *not* like that.

Think of all the things you buy or rent that have a posted price that you know before the purchase: everything at the grocery store, restaurant meals, gas, cars, computers, phones, clothing, houses, legal and other professional fees, Uber rides, hotel rooms, airline tickets, furniture, toys, insurance, boats.... almost everything. I can't think of anything we buy that we don't know the price beforehand, except for healthcare. OK, I thought of one: auctions (and even they often have a posted minimum bid).

Admittedly, you don't always pay the posted price, but never more than that. Even for repair work, such as on cars, you can usually get a ballpark estimate in advanced (enforceable by law in some jurisdictions). Some legal and other professional fees can be tricky due to the inherent open-ended nature of the business. For instance, I am employed as a hospitalist. My employer should be able to tell my patients what they charge for a hospital admission and daily daily follow-up visit. What we don't know is how long you'll be in the hospital.

We desperately need healthcare price transparency.

What's the best thing about healthcare price transparency? It turns 270,000,000 U.S. adults into price-conscious consumers of healthcare. This immediately increases competition in the marketplace as providers start to compete for business partially on the basis of price. As it is now, once the insurance deductible is met, someone other than the patient is paying for healthcare.

And that someone may not give a damn how much something costs because they'll simply pass that cost on to the patient or employer. E.g., higher insurance premiums or deductibles next year.

My very first accountant in Austin, TX, seared into my brain that "no one cares about your money as much as you do." The money your employer pays for your health insurance premiums is money that your worked earned. If not going to the insurance company, it would be yours.

Price transparency also might, just might, shame some of the healthcare price-gougers into lowering their prices. Consumers could easily find out that Hospital A charges patients $1 for an aspirin tablet while Hospital B charges $17. Hospital B has some 'splainin' to do.

The American Hospital Association doesn't seem to be in favor of price transparency:

From *The New York Times* in 2019 (49):

> The nation's hospital groups sued the Trump administration on Wednesday over a new federal rule [Hospital Price Transparency Rule] that would require them to disclose the discounted prices they give insurers for all sorts of procedures.
>
> The hospitals, including the American Hospital Association, **argued in a lawsuit** filed in United States District Court in Washington that the new rule "is unlawful, several times over."
>
> They argued that the administration exceeded its legal authority in **issuing the rule last month** as part of its efforts to make the health care system much more transparent to patients. The lawsuit contends the

requirement to disclose their private negotiations with insurers violates their First Amendment rights.

"We make the case that the burden placed on our members to come up with this information is extensive," Tom Nickels, an executive vice president with the American Hospital Association, said in an interview.

I'm not sure how that lawsuit turned out but according to *Health Affairs* (86), a federal rule went into effect in July, 2021, requiring *hospitals* to reveal negotiated prices for all items and services. Similarly, a federal rule in July, 2022, requires *health plans* to disclose the negotiated prices they pay facilities and physicians for all items and services they provide.

From *Health Affairs*:

> With the **primary goal** of improving consumer decision making, the Centers for Medicare and Medicaid Services (CMS) issued rules requiring both hospitals and insurers to make their negotiated prices public….Hospitals now have to publish the following in a machine-readable format for all the items and services they provide: gross charges, discounted cash price for those not using insurance, payer-specific negotiated prices, de-identified minimum negotiated price, and de-identified maximum negotiated price. Hospitals are also required to prominently, publicly, and in "plain language," display their prices for 300 of the most commonly used services, as defined by CMS.

How good is compliance by hospitals and insurers? Again, from *Health Affairs*:

> Hospitals have been slow to comply with transparency

rules. Between July and September 2021, fewer than 6 percent of hospitals had disclosed prices as required. Hospitals with higher revenues and in highly consolidated markets were found to be more likely to flout the law. CMS has set a maximum fine of about $2 million a year for larger hospitals that fail to comply, but some of these hospitals have stated that they would rather pay the fines than forgo their competitive advantage. As of June 2022, CMS has issued 352 warning notices and 157 corrective action plan requests to hospitals. CMS has also fined two hospitals in Georgia; the fines amounted to only 0.04 percent of the hospitals' net patient revenue.

Even when hospitals have complied with the rules, experts have found the data to be "consistently inconsistent" in terms of how data elements are defined and displayed, making it very difficult for third parties to make connections across hospitals and payers. Based on their experience with hospital transparency rules, CMS issued several pieces of technical guidance to insurers before the rules applicable to health plans went into effect. Insurers that fail to comply with health plan transparency rules will face fines of around $100 per violation, per day, per affected enrollee, which can quickly add up to far larger fines than those faced by hospitals. Initial reports suggest that most insurers have complied with the technical requirements of the rule, but the data files they have posted are largely inaccessible and indecipherable to anyone without access to a supercomputer.

A study published in 2023 (94) found that only 25% of the nation's largest health system hospitals were in complete compliance with the Hospital Price

Transparency Rule

The drug companies, for their part, definitely aren't if favor of price transparency. They want you to assume drugs are expensive all over the world. They want you to think that without high prices, they'd stop innovating and discovering new or better drugs.

2. THIRD PARTY INTERFERENCE IN THE PATIENT-PROVIDER RELATIONSHIP

Third parties are mostly insurance companies, government, Big Pharma, and managed care organizations (MCOs, which are often insurance companies themselves). None of these third parties work for free. Who's paying them? You. And you're not getting your money's worth.

Let's tackle insurance interference first. The health insurance market is now so distorted that many of us have forgotten what insurance is. *True or traditional insurance* is a bet. You're betting a small amount of money (the premium) that something bad, very expensive, and relatively *rare* is going to happen to you. (You don't want to win that bet but as we all know, "shit happens.") The insurance company takes the other side of that bet, figuring the rare bad thing won't happen to you, so they can keep your premium dollars, Of course, that premium must include dollars for administrative costs and some profit.

Take term life insurance, for example. You're betting (your insurance premium) that you're going to die within the next 10 years, and when you do, your designated survivor (e.g., your spouse) gets $250,000. The insurance company is betting that you won't die, in which case the insurance company keeps all of the monthly premiums you paid for the last ten years. If you're a healthy 25-year-old man, it's not at all likely you'll die before you're 35, so your monthly premium is only $20. On the other hand, if you're an overweight 65-year-old with hypertension and diabetes, you're much more likely to die within the next ten years, so your monthly premium is $250.

If you're 25-years-old with a wife and baby, but zero or negative net worth, paying $20/month for the life insurance is reasonable. On the other hand, the 65-year-old with net worth of $2 million probably won't make that bet at $250/month. When he dies, his survivor(s) get his $2 million. How much premium you're willing to pay depends on your risk tolerance.

Understand that the insurance company has loads of money, so their risk tolerance is extremely high. They even have their own insurance just in case they have losses that exceed their available cash. They have experts that calculate the odds of a bad thing happening, which is also informed by their past experience. They already have a very good idea how many healthy 25-year-old men will die within 10 years. The premium they charge reflects that knowledge, plus extra administrative expenses and profit. Don't worry about the insurance companies; they're doing OK.

Other examples of *true insurance* that make sense for middle-class people would be homeowner's insurance and liability insurance for people who drive. In these instances, there's a small probability of a large loss that would wipe you out financially.

In contrast to true or traditional insurance, *fake insurance* is characterized as "I'll have somebody else pay my bills for me." An example is federally-subsidized flood insurance, subsidized by taxpayer dollars. Some homes are intentionally built on flood-prone areas such as beaches or river flood plains. They are going to flood every five, ten, or hundred years. Oh, but the views! True insurance for those homes should be very expensive, but the owners of those properties have powerful friends, so the whole country has to subsidize their insurance. "Insurance" like this is better labelled as federal spending.

Health insurance in the U.S. is almost always the fake "*you* pay my bills" insurance. Premiums of the young and healthy pay bills of the old and sick, men pay the bills of women, wealthy or insured patients pay for the uninsured and indigents. We've gotten to the point where many folks can't tell the difference between protection from rare risks and somebody else paying their bills. If health insurance simply covered rare yet expensive events, it would be easy to afford. Some more examples fake insurance:

- Small and routine expenses like doctor visits and oral contraceptives are covered by insurance. Since these are not rare and expensive events, the cost is just preloaded into your premium, which includes a percentage for the insurance company's trouble. So you pay more than if you simply paid from your own pocket.

- Pre-existing conditions in the past were not covered by insurance, for the same reason that you can't but term insurance when you're bedridden with terminal cancer. Since passage of the Affordable Care Act, pre-existing conditions are covered, and the government had to kick in more money to insurance companies in order for it to make financial sense.

- Women of child-bearing age have much higher medical expenses than men, especially if they get pregnant, but since passage of the Affordable Care Act it is illegal to charge women a higher premium than men.

There are basically two types of health insurance in America today: managed care organizations and private fee-for-service (also known as indemnity).

The indemnity sector has shrunk to 10-15% of the insurance market. Indemnity insurance is what folks had before managed care rose to prominence, and came in either Basic or Major Medical packages. If you had this type of insurance, you would typically pay for your medical care out-of-pocket then file a claim with the insurance company for re-imbursement (which is "indemnification"). Or the healthcare provider might submit the claim for you. Back when indemnity insurance was dominant, healthcare dollars as a percentage of gross domestic product was much lower. For example, the percentage of GDP devoted to healthcare was 5% in 1960 (61). The law establishing Medicare was passed in 1965. By 1968, the GDP healthcare percentage was up to 6%. The Health Maintenance Organization Act creating managed care organizations passed in 1973. And by 1976, the healthcare GDP percentage was up to 8%. I wouldn't blame you for thinking the federal government carries some blame for rising healthcare costs. I certainly do. But there are alternate possibilities. It's complicated. Some would argue that without government involvement, the increases would have been even higher. Here we are in 2024 with the percentage of GDP chewed up by healthcare now over three times higher than in 1960.

Managed care organizations (MCOs) were created by the Health Maintenance Organization Act of 1973. The HMO Act was a response to concern about rising healthcare costs. (Fun Fact: Medicare was started in 1965, just eight years before the HMO Act. Hmmm...wonder if Medicare is related to rising healthcare costs.) Eighty to 90% of American workers are enrolled in managed care organizations. Increasing numbers of Medicaid and Medicare patients are also covered by MCOs.

MCOs may solely manage healthcare benefits of enrollees. Perhaps more often, MCOs are also insurance companies, or act like insurers.

The main types of MCOs are:

- HMO: health maintenance organization
- PPO: preferred provider organization (the most common MCO)
- POS: point of service organization
- EPO: exclusive provider organization
- PHO: physician-hospital organization
- ACO: accountable care organization (introduced by Obamacare)

In their efforts to hold down costs, managed care organizations can utilize a variety of options, including:

- High deductibles (four in 10 adults in the U.S. under age 65 are on high-deductible insurance plans)
- Intensive oversight and management of high-cost diseases and patients
- Review of healthcare utilization by providers and patients
- Negotiate discount prices from providers
- Restrict access to medical specialists
- Incentivize (think $) physicians and patients to choose less costly care
- Incentivize physicians to follow the MCO's medical guidelines
- Require prior authorization for high-cost care
- Emphasize preventative care and wellness

Those cost-containment efforts require lots of clerks and administrators, aka bureaucrats. They don't work for free and are one reason healthcare is so expensive in the U.S. Fun Fact: In French, "bureau" means desk.

There is lively debate among the experts whether MCOs have tamped down healthcare costs or altered the overall quality of care over the last several decades.

Federal and state governments are also meddlesome third-parties in the patient-provider relationship.

Take EMTALA, for instance. Passed in 1986, the Emergency Medical Treatment and Labor Act requires every Medicare-participating hospital (that's nearly all of them) to provide a medical screening exam for everyone that shows up at the Emergency Department, regardless of ability to pay for services. If a true emergency condition is present, the hospital is required to stabilize it, which may require admission or transfer to a higher level of care. Sounds great, doesn't it?

Before we get into the problems posed by EMTALA, let's look at emergency department charges. Emergency department charges are usually 5 to 10 times higher than non-emergency care at a physician office or urgent care center. For instance, if you show up at an emergency department with a headache or abdominal pain, you almost always will get blood tests done plus head CT scan or abdominal-pelvic CT scan. CT scans are expensive. Take the same headache or abdominal pain to your PCP's office, and Dr Jayasankar, if she's a good clinician, can diagnose you by just talking to you and examining you 90% of the time, no CT scan needed. (The belly pain will require some blood tests, and perhaps imaging studies later.)

Here are some problems with EMTALA. It's not always clear what constitutes an "emergency condition." It's not always clear what "stabilization" means. The general public knows they cannot be turned down for evaluation by an emergency department due to lack of ability to pay, so many folks show up with issues that aren't emergencies, such as ingrown toenails, sprained ankles, head colds, tension headaches, and poison ivy. Emergency departments know there are heavy fines and potential banishment from the Medicare program if they make a mistake in terms of "emergency condition" or "stabilization." So they typically accept all comers as true emergencies, evaluating and treating everyone. To compensate for folks who can't pay for "emergency" care, emergency department charges are raised for those who have insurance or otherwise can pay for care. So insured and wealthy folks are subsidizing the others who may have chosen to spend money on cigarettes, alcohol, vacations, bass boats, cable TV, Netflix, or cellphones. There's a lot of over-use of emergency departments by folks who don't have emergencies or don't have access to office-based care. Or they just don't want to wait for an office appointment. This over-use is difficult to quantify in dollars. Making office-based care more affordable and accessible will help alleviate this problem.

You probably haven't heard of a third-party called HEDIS (Healthcare Effectiveness Data and Information Set). Yet the NCQA (National Committee for Quality Assurance) website says 191 million people are enrolled in plans that report HEDIS results. Medicare, for example, requires their approved health plans to participate. HEDIS (53) is ostensibly a performance improvement tool. HEDIS measures include:

- Effectiveness of care
- Access/availability of care
- Utilization
- Risk adjusted utilization
- Measures collected using electronic clinical data systems

See reference (54) for details on approximately 90 health plan performance measures. NCQA, who owns HEDIS, may be doing great things to improve quality of care in the U.S. Or not. I don't know. But I do know they don't work for free. Someone's paying for their overhead expenses, software, and the data entry clerks at the healthcare plans that report to NCQA. The program undoubtedly contributes to the cost of healthcare. If done right, NCQA and HEDIS could reduce the cost of healthcare or improve health outcomes, but I've not seen evidence for that.

Another way the government interferes in the patient-physician relationship is in fee setting, addressed in the next section.

Another area of third-party interference by the government is insurance benefit mandates, and there are thousands of them (55). I.e., government requires you to buy specific coverage that you don't want or don't need. This will vary state by state, while the federal Affordable Care Act established 10 mandates that apply to all individual plans and small group plans. They might include sex-change operations, birth control, maternity services, infertility treatments, drug and alcohol treatment programs, coverage for pre-existing conditions, to name a few. Economist James Bailey notes that in 1970 the average state had less than one mandated benefit, but by 2011 the average state had 37 mandates (56). He calculated that **new mandates were responsible for 9 to 23% of all premium increases over the 1996-2011 period.** Healthcare cost savings by eliminating certain benefit mandates will vary from state to state and are difficult to calculate. If a state demands coverage for something you don't want or need, it means you're subsidizing other folks who want that coverage. Is that fair? Why not let individual consumers choose and pay for the benefits they want? In 2024, Liberty Mutual insurance company was running TV ads that say, "We customize your car insurance so you only pay for what you need!" Insurance mandates prevent you from doing that with health insurance.

A major problem with third parties is that they usually

don't care about the cost of care. They've got no "skin in the game." Especially if they can simply pass higher costs on to the enrollees or employers via higher premiums, higher deductibles, or taxes.

3. GOVERNMENT FEE SETTING

Like all businesses, healthcare providers always have what are called "overhead expenses." They have to pay these to open and run a business. Things like rent or mortgage payments, electric and water bills, support staff salaries, insurance, phone service, equipment, furniture, etc. Providers must set the fees they charge at a level that covers all their overhead costs plus some profit for the owner to live on. In all successful free-market businesses, prices for services are set at a level to cover overhead expenses plus some profit. Admittedly, the profit portion is usually as high as the market will bear, reflecting 1) supply and demand, and 2) competition in the marketplace. But without profit, there is no business. Without profit, there is no business. Period.

Total U.S. healthcare spending in 2022 was $4.5 trillion, or ~$13,500 per person. Public health insurance programs like Medicare and Medicaid spend 39% of all healthcare dollars (57). To hospitals and physicians, Medicare and Medicaid pay only 50 to 80% of the amount other insurers pay for care rendered. This is one reason you may have trouble finding a provider who wants to treat you if you have Medicare or Medicaid. If the pay is too low, the provider loses money. And providers doing lots of that won't stay in business long. When I worked in Florida in the 1990s, I knew a physician who didn't even bother to bill Medicaid; the pay was so low it wasn't worth the trouble. If a provider does see Medicare and Medicaid patients for marginal or non-existent profit, they have to jack the prices up for other patients. Why doesn't the government just pay a fair price for services? Or at least make systemic changes that lower the healthcare provider's overhead costs? Then at some point, a marginal payment becomes profitable.

If you want to employ the professional services of an attorney, accountant, interior designer, real estate agent, or home remodeler, the professional tells you the fee he has set. You can agree, negotiate, or move on to another professional. In contrast, in 1992 Medicare established its non-negotiable physician fee schedule. In other words, if Dr Desai "opted-in" and participated in the Medicare program, she would accept whatever Medicare decided was fair pay for her services. The fee was based partially on what Medicare figured the doc's overhead cost was. For instance, urban physicians got paid more than rural. Most physicians then (and now) participated in the Medicare program.

One problem with the government fee schedule is that the worst physician or provider in town is paid the very same for service as the very best physician or provider. (This may change due to the MACRA program. Said program has its own problems, including high administrative costs to the provider.) Let's say the service is a groin hernia repair. The worst surgeon has a high rate of surgical site infections, a high rate of needing a second operation at the same site, and a high-than-average rate of deaths within 30 days after operation. The best surgeon has the opposite of all that, plus glowing reviews on social media. Medicare pays each surgeon the same amount for the operation. Other than malpractice lawsuits, what's to motivate the poor surgeon to improve his game? What's to motivate the great surgeon to work hard to get even better? It won't be his pay rate, that's for sure. So this government pay scheme promotes mediocrity and inhibits innovation. If you want to improve healthcare, you must financially reward competent and successful competitors. A pat on the back and an "atta boy" are not enough reward. Certainly not enough for a new physician who has $200,000 of medical school debt to pay back (58).

4. EXCESSIVE ADMINISTRATIVE COSTS

Administrative costs are inescapable. They are the nonclinical costs of running a medical system. The primary components are 1) billing and insurance-related (BIR), and 2) hospital or physician practice administration. Billing and insurance-related expenses are about half of administrative costs in the U.S., and refer to the overhead costs for the insurance industry, and provider costs for claims submission, payment processing, and claim reconciliation. The Center for American Progress estimates that the total spending on BIR in 2019 was $496 million. They cite a 2010 estimate by the National Academy of Medicine that the U.S. spends twice as much as necessary on BIR.

Research on administrative costs is difficult to do, and you'll find estimates all over the map, from 8.3% to 34% of total U.S healthcare costs (41, 42, 43, 44). The true cost is likely somewhere between those extremes, toward the higher end. If you look into the literature, be sure you're comparing apples to apples. Using the same methodology to compare the U.S. to other high-income OECD countries, the U.S. spent twice as much-8.3% of health spending-as the average of the other countries. The experts agree that the U.S.is #1 in administrative expenses. But why pay more than is necessary?

A 2021 report (2) published by The Commonwealth Fund ranked the U.S. #11 in Administrative Efficiency among 11 high-income OECD countries. The other countries in the study, listed from most to least efficient, were Norway, Australia, New Zealand, UK, Sweden, France, Canada, Netherlands, Germany, and Switzerland.

Physician offices, hospitals, and healthcare systems employ legions of clerks and administrators to produce and file insurance claims, process payments, appeal denied claims, and navigate the nuances of multiple insurance contracts. None of this provides direct care and comfort to patients.

Insurance companies employ their own armies of clerks and administrators to process the aforementioned insurance claims, including denial of payment as often as they can. None of this provides direct care and comfort to patients.

Managed Care Organizations also do much of the claims processing as above, plus monitor and enforce compliance of providers to the terms of their contracts. For instance, is Dr Lolabhattu prescribing generics instead of brand-name drugs? Is Dr Shah prescribing the particular statin drug on the "approved-drugs list" (aka formulary) instead of one of the other six on the market? Dr Shah doesn't know we changed our approved statin two weeks ago! "Doctor Aggarwal, that lumbar MRI scan doesn't meet our criteria for medical necessity. I'll email you the guideline." "I'm sorry, but we only allow eight physical therapy sessions every six months and you've already used those." "We can't approve the wheelchair request until you've documented failure of crutches, canes, and rolling walkers first. Please submit appropriate documentation." "Dr Gupta, you're only seeing 20 office patients a day. Your peers are averaging 27. You'll have to pick up the pace." None of this provides direct care and comfort to patients.

Public health insurers, e.g., Medicare and Medicaid, or their contracted intermediaries also employ numerous clerks and administrators to process claims and ensure compliance with their programs.

5. LOBBYING

Lobbying is an attempt by individuals or organizations to influence legislation and policy at the federal, state, or local level. It's not a bad thing per se. It's not illegal. In addition to in-person visits with legislators, lobbying often involves gifts, campaign contributions, mutual back-scratching, or bribes to the legislators or their family, friends, or business associates. Some of this is, or should be, illegal.

If you or your organization don't have much money or celebrity, you won't make any headway influencing governmental policy, particularly at higher levels of government. You may not even get a five-minute meeting with your representative. Money talks, malarkey walks. Your rulers consider your issue malarkey if you have no money.

The examples of big-money influence on legislation and regulation are legion. For one example, check out "How healthcare's Washington lobbying machine gets the job done" at *Modern Healthcare* magazine (16). You'll learn how much expensive lobbying it cost for Gilead Sciences to get approval of their hepatitis C drug, Sovaldi. You'll learn about the incestuous revolving door among industry, Congressional staffers and policy advisors, retired politicians and regulators, and trade or professional associations:

> In 2011 and 2012, the company spent just under $3 million on lobbying, according to reports. Last year, that figure increased to just over $4 million, a jump of more than 40%. And through the first two quarters of 2014, the company spent $2.6 million on lobbying, putting it on track to top $5 million for the year.

Open Secrets (17) reported that the healthcare industry spent $739 million on federal lobbying in 2023. Of that total, $379 million was lobbying on behalf of drugs and health products, $131 million for hospitals and nursing homes, and $120 million for healthcare services and HMOs.

Statista (87) produced a list of the leading lobbying industries in the U.S. in 2022: Leading the pack was pharmaceuticals/health products at $373 million. Far behind at #2 was electronics manufacturing & equipment at $221 million. #7 was hospitals/nursing homes at $124 million. #10 was health services/HMOs at $122 million. #15 was health professionals at $96 million. In case you're wondering, positions 3 through 6 were insurance, securities & investment, real estate, and business associations, respectively.

A January 2020 article at Axios by Bob Herman details the amount of money ($309 million) spent on federal lobbying by 60 of the largest U.S. healthcare companies and trade organizations in 2019 (47).

The article lists the top 20 spenders on lobbying in 2019:

1. Pharmaceutical Research and Manufacturers of America (aka PhRMA): $28,900,000

2. American Hospital Association: $22,160,000

3. American Medical Association: $20,030,000

4. Biotechnology Innovation Organization (trade association for drugs/devices companies): $12,210,000

5. Pfizer (drugs/devices): $10,990,000

6. Amgen (drugs/devices): $10,940,000

7. America's Health Insurance Plans (insurers): $9,540,000

8. CVS Health/Aetna (Aetna health insurance, pharmacies, MinuteClinics, pharmacy benefits management): $9,487,000

9. Genentech (biotech pharmaceuticals): $8,690,000

10. Cigna/Express Scripts (health insurance/pharmacy benefits management): $8,250,000

11. Merck (drugs, vaccines): $6,955,000

12. Eli Lilly (drugs/devices): $6,910,000

13. Blue Cross Blue Shield Association (insurers):

$6,840,000

14. AbbVie (drugs): $6,340,000

15. Novartis (drugs/devices): $5,970,000

16. Johnson & Johnson (drugs/devices, consumer products): $5,750,000

17. Gilead Sciences (drugs): $5,720,000

18. Humana (health insurance, administers Medicare Advantage programs and Tricare): $5,690,000

19. Sanofi (drugs): $5,117,000

20. Anthem (health insurance, pharmacy benefits manager, administers Medicare Advantage programs): $5,070,000

The pharmaceutical industry spent more than other industries and trade organizations. Many of the individual drug companies listed also contribute to the #1 spender, PhRMA.

These figures don't include campaign contributions, trade association dues, or state-level lobbying.

Here's an example of lobbying published by The National Bureau of Economic Research (15):

> We study the interplay between congressional politics and health care spending in the U.S. by examining events leading up to and following the passage of the 2003 Medicare Modernization Act (MMA). The MMA, which Congress narrowly approved, created prescription drug coverage for seniors. We focus on a provision in the law - Section 508 - which allowed hospitals to apply for Medicare payment increases

that were awarded based on rules written after the MMA was passed. This paper provides evidence of a feedback loop that illustrates why provisions, like Section 508, which are common, get added to laws, raise spending, and then become exceedingly hard to eliminate. We present evidence that the Section 508 program was used to win political support for the MMA. We find that Representatives who voted 'Yea' to the MMA were more likely to have a hospital in their district awarded a Section 508 waiver. The Section 508 program led to large increases in health spending (approximately 18 percent at treated hospitals) and the creation of hundreds of local jobs. The Section 508 program was slated to expire three years after it was introduced. However, millions were spent lobbying to extend the program. After the program was extended, we observe that members of Congress with recipient-hospitals in their district received large increases in campaign contributions. Ultimately, the marginal increase in health spending generated by the Section 508 program dramatically exceeded what Congress initially authorized for the program and dwarfed the amount spent on lobbying to extend the program.

I was not able to find a reliable estimate of how much total money is spent on combined federal and state healthcare lobbying. I think the medical-industrial complex wants it that way. With a little digging, you may be able to find out how much is spent on healthcare lobbying in your state. For instance, in Vermont in 2018, the healthcare industry was the highest spender on statehouse lobbying at $1.8 million, nearly twice as much as the second highest-spending sector: energy (18).

6. INADEQUATE INCENTIVE TO GET AND STAY HEALTHY

Only 20% of U.S. adults and adolescents are doing enough exercise to maximize health and longevity.

How much exercise does it take? The Department of Health and Human Services recommends that adults do 150 to 300 minutes of moderate-intensity exercise or 75 to 150 minutes of vigorous-intensity physical activity each week, along with at least two days a week of muscle-strengthening exercises.

One-third of U.S. adults are obese (body mass index over 30; use an online calculator to determine your BMI). Here's a laundry list of obesity-related conditions to remind you why you want to avoid obesity, or reverse it:

- Premature death. It starts at BMI of 30, with a major increase in premature death at BMI over 40. The U.S. has 200,000 yearly deaths directly attributable to obesity.

- Arthritis, especially of the knees.

- Type 2 diabetes mellitus. Eighty-five percent of people with type 2 diabetes are overweight or obese.

- Increased cardiovascular disease risk, especially with an apple-shaped body fat distribution as compared to pear-shaped. Cardiovascular disease includes heart attacks, high blood pressure, strokes, and peripheral arterial disease (poor circulation).

- Obstructive sleep apnea.

- Gallstones are three or four times more common in the obese.

- High blood pressure. At least one third of cases are caused by excess body fat. Every 20 pounds of excess fat raises blood pressure 2-3 points (mmHg).

- Tendency to higher total and LDL cholesterol, higher triglycerides, while lowering HDL cholesterol. These lipid changes are associated with hardening of the arteries – atherosclerosis – which can lead to heart attacks, strokes, and peripheral arterial disease.

- Increased cancers. Prostate and colorectal in men. Endometrial, gallbladder, cervix, ovary, and breast in women. Kidney and esophageal adenocarcinoma in both sexes. Excess fat contributes to 14-20% of all cancer-related deaths in the U.S. Over 550,000 people die from cancer in the U.S. yearly. Twenty percent of us will die from cancer.

- Strokes.

- Low back pain.

- Gout.

- Varicose veins.

- Hemorrhoids.

- Blood clots in legs and lungs.

- Surgery complications: poor wound healing, blood clots, wound infection, breathing problems.

- Pregnancy complications: toxemia, high blood pressure, diabetes, prolonged labor, greater need for C-section.

- Fat build-up in liver.

- Asthma.

- Low sperm counts.

- Decreased fertility.

- Delayed or missed diagnosis due to difficult physical examination or weight exceeding the limit of diagnostic equipment.

Trust me, I'm a doctor. Adequate exercise and avoidance or reversal of obesity will go a long way to keeping us healthy and out of the clutches of the medical-industrial complex. We'll spend less money on healthcare, too!

But how do we motivate folks to exercise and control weight, while preventing health problems that may not manifest in the individual until 20 years hence? I've been pondering that for decades of medical practice and have no definite answers. Heck, I need to lose 15 pounds and exercise more myself. There are no inducements that work for everyone at all times. The strongest motivator is a serious health scare personally or in a loved one.

Here are a few ideas for promoting a healthy lifestyle....

1. Ongoing education of the public. I'm not very optimistic about this because it hasn't been very

successful over the last half decade. But there are glimmers of hope. Cigarette smokers dropped by 68 percent among U.S. adults, from 43 percent in 1965 to 14 percent in 2018. Education put the fear of lung cancer and chronic lung disease into smokers. Emotions like fear seem to be more motivational than rationality. Doesn't everybody already know that regular exercise and healthy body weights keep us healthier over the long run? But a commitment to that is harder than quitting cigarettes.

2.   Money is another good motivator for some folks. Remember a TV show called "The Biggest Loser"? It was a competition among obese players to see who could lose the most weight in the span of 30 weeks, typically via brutal exercise and calorie restriction. In the early years, the winner was awarded $250,000. Competition was fierce. If you needed to lose 100 lb of excess weight over the next year, would $250,000 motivate you? But nobody's going to pay you that, nor $100,000, not even $10,000.

Smaller scale Biggest Loser-style competitions could be done in physician offices, commercial gyms, company offices, and churches. Have contestants pay a $100 entry fee to cover administrative costs and the prize money. It doesn't have to be winner-take-all. Second and third place awards are motivational, too. It wouldn't be fair to have someone needing to lose 15 pounds compete with someone who needs to lose 150. There are other ways to set it up, with a little imagination. You may not even have to offer a cash prize. (I'm well aware that most of the winners and losers in the TV show quickly regained lost weight. I don't advocate dramatic rapid weight loss.)

3.   What if you got a significant discount on health

insurance premiums or a lower deductible if you demonstrated a certain level of fitness on a yearly treadmill or stationary bicycle stress test? You'd save the insurer money over time; they should share that with you. The biggest losers are the healthcare providers who will see you less often. On a related note, I recently met a patient who mentioned that her insurer pays her a small amount every month if she if she walks a certain number of average daily steps.

4. High-deductible health insurance pressures consumers to stay as healthy as possible when they're paying for the first few thousands of dollars for care.

In a way, having health insurance is a perverse incentive to be lackadaisical about your health. Like, "I've got great insurance that'll come in handy if I get sick, so I'm not gonna worry about getting and staying healthy now."

It's possible the high cost of healthcare has induced some folks to get and stay healthier. We know it has discouraged many from seeking necessary healthcare.

5. Have you heard that walking 10,000 steps a day may will improve your longevity? 10,000 steps is roughly five miles, depending on your stride length. If that seems daunting, the latest research (88) suggests that 6,000-8,000 steps may be just as effective, depending on your age. And if you're an older woman (average age 72), 4,400 steps may be enough (89).

7. INADEQUATE COMPETITION

Most products and services compete on the basis of price and quality. Those features are usually mysteries in the healthcare sector.

As it is now, the price of a medical service or product to a consumer depends on payment type (cash versus insurance), the insurance deductible amount and whether it's been met for the year, whether the provider is in-network or out-of-network, the place of service (clinic, hospital, urgent care, emergency department), whether someone from the billing office is available to tell you the price (not available on weekends and nights), whether your prescription is on the insurer's formulary, whether you could find an online discount for your prescription, etc. In other words, we rarely have price transparency. Clear and readily available prices are necessary to improve competition based on price.

Quality comparisons are a harder nut to crack. Online product and service reviews are not ideal but are a piece of the puzzle. If you're looking for a physician, ask other physicians who they would see or send their relatives to. Nurses and pharmacists may also have solid recommendations. Ask friends and relatives which provider they had a good experience with. But remember that a good experience does not necessarily equal good care. If you know a personal injury lawyer who does malpractice cases, they should know names of both the excellent and bad local doctors. If you're having a procedure done, use a provider who's done a lot of them. If you're having open heart surgery, use a hospital that does 200 a year rather than 20 a year. A provider with five years' experience is likely to be better than one fresh out of training. You may be able to check out your prospective provider at a state medical or other licensing board. Lots of complaints filed? Any disciplinary action taken? You may be able to search online county or state court records to see if your provider has been sued often. Licensing board complaints and lawsuits don't necessarily indicate bad care, but are puzzle pieces. You need to change providers if yours is too rushed, doesn't listen to you, doesn't communicate well, has rude office staff, or is disrespectful of your time. Can we create something like Underwriters Laboratories (https://ul.org) for healthcare providers and products?

As mentioned elsewhere in this document, we need to financially reward the better healthcare providers. Unlike Medicare paying the worst and best physician in town the same fee.

The next example could also be filed under Excessive Regulation below. But it's also anti-competitive. I'm talking about the con job that is CON: certificates of need. For example, say you want to build a hospital in a specific area and think you can compete successfully against the other hospitals there. You build your hospital and the marketplace determines whether you'll be successful or not, right? Wrong, at least in many parts of the country (90). Many states require you to obtain a certificate of need from bureaucrats before you can build your hospital. Do you think other hospitals in the area welcome the competition? They don't. Do you think other hospitals might try to influence the bureaucrats and politicians to put the kibosh on your plans? They will. Multi-millions of dollars in profit are at play in deals like this. Consider this excerpt from an un-dated (probably 2006) *Birmingham Medical News* article (19):

> In Alabama, a former governor has just been convicted of selling a seat on the state Certificate of Need

Review Board in exchange for donations. Meanwhile, Louisiana, which dropped its CON program two decades ago after its governor was accused of selling hospital permits, finished up a legislative session that did little to advance healthcare reform in the state, including a failed bill that would have set up a CON review process in the rebuilding of New Orleans' hospitals.

Certificate of need programs date back to 1974, when Congress set up the system in an attempt to contain healthcare costs. It was repealed in 1986. Twenty years later, there's still no clear-cut answer as to the benefits of these programs. CON programs still exist in about two-thirds of the states, including Alabama. Other states, such as Louisiana, have done away with them.

In 2004, The Federal Trade Commission and the Department of Justice issued a report concluding that CON does not control healthcare costs and is used to create barriers to competition. At the same time, there's mixed evidence on whether CON affects quality of care.

***

....Alabama is one of the few states that still has a politically appointed review committee, with each new governor appointing a new CON review board. That offers potential for corruption. Former Gov. Don Siegelman and HealthSouth founder Richard Scrushy were convicted in late June on charges that Scrushy bought a seat on the board in exchange for $500,000 in contributions.

Did you know the federal government keeps a record of

medical malpractice lawsuits that resulted in financial judgements or settlements involving certain providers such as physicians? It's the National Practitioner Data Bank. Your tax dollars pay for it but you can't access it. Would that information help you choose a physician? Releasing that information to the public would be pro-competitive.

8. EXCESSIVE DRUG COSTS

Patients shouldn't have to choose between taking a life-saving drug and paying their electric bill.

Spending on prescription drugs in the U.S. accounted for 9% of total healthcare costs in 2022 (59). And that doesn't include your non-prescription drugs like Tylenol, Nyquil, and Advil. Annual pharmaceutical spending per capita in the U.S. in 2022 was $1,432 compared to a range of $402 to $1,042 in other high-income countries (91). Cancer drugs are typically priced at $120,000 to $150,000 per year, some of which only extend life another couple months. At least one former pharmaceutical executive (13) has admitted that the price of medicines isn't based on research and development costs, "... **it is determined by their value in preventing and treating disease.**"

We in the U.S. spent $405,900,000,000 on prescription drugs in 2022 (59). Let's round that off to $406 billion.

Drugs are so expensive here that many folks make trips to Canada and Mexico for major savings. Or they use online pharmacies based abroad. While both are technically illegal under federal law, prosecutions seem to be rare, at least for those who aren't re-selling the drugs here.

Be aware that development of new drugs is extremely expensive. Millions of dollars, by some estimates over a billion. Most promising new drugs turn out to be duds and never make it to market. Pharmaceutical companies that take the risk of drug development deserve to be compensated with profit. Unfortunately for U.S. consumers, much of that profit comes from the U.S. market rather than worldwide. Successful drugs are sold in other nations generally at a significantly reduced price compared to the U.S. That's not fair. For instance, scorpion sting antivenom in the U.S. costs thousands of dollars whereas in Mexico it's in the hundreds.

In general, the length of a drug patent in the U.S. is 20 years from the date of patent application. The patent protects the investment of the drug developer. Another protection for the drug developer is "exclusivity." Exclusivity refers to certain delays and prohibitions on approval of competitor drugs available under the statute that attach upon approval of a drug or of certain supplements (51).

Brand-name drugs that are under patent protection are generally more expensive than the generic versions of those drugs that are available after expiration of the patent. Pharmaceutical companies have been known to pay a generic manufacturer to postpone production for a while, thus maintaining the higher price of the brand-name drug. Yes, that's legal.

Big Pharma executives say that without the potential pay-off of successful patented drugs, they couldn't continue to fund their life-saving research. Guess who's the biggest single funder of drug research and development.

It's you. The U.S taxpayer via the National Institutes of Health (NIH) in 2017 spent $32 billion versus the $71 billion from all the members of PhRMA, the primary pharmaceutical industry lobbying organization (12). (The cited article implies that the $32 billion from NIH was purely drug research but I suppose it could be all health-related research.) I wouldn't be surprised if the industry spends as much or more on sales and marketing as they do on research and development. A more recent analysis (107) found that "the magnitude of NIH investment in new drugs is comparable with that of the industry..." This study, published at JAMA Network in 2023, looked at NIH versus industry funding of 356 new drugs approved by the FDA between 2010 and 2019. Researchers found that "spending from the NIH was not less than industry funding." (Yes, that's odd phrasing.) The NIH spent $1.44 billion per approval on basic or applied research for products with novel targets or $599 million per approval considering applications of basic research to multiple products. From the report's Discussion section:

These analyses suggest that NIH project costs for basic or applied research associated with the products approved from 2010 to 2019 were significantly greater than reported industry spending. Costs for the NIH were also higher than industry costs when both included spending on failed clinical trials of candidate products. Including clinical failures, NIH investment (calculated with either a 3% or 7% discount rate) was not less than industry investment calculated with a 10.5% cost of capital. Investment from the NIH calculated with clinical failures and a 3% or 7% discount rate was also not less than industry investment calculated with clinical failures, additional costs of prehuman research, and 10.5% cost of capital. These results suggest that NIH investments in pharmaceutical innovation are comparable with those made by industry.

Have you heard of Pharmacy Benefit Management companies (PBMs) or Group Purchasing Organizations? PBMs are difficult to explain. I've spent two or three hours trying to figure them out and still don't fully understand how they work. For extra credit, see references (71), (72, especially Exhibit 1 Powerpoint slide), and (73). First off, keep in mind that PBMs work for the health insurers; in many cases they are *owned* by the insurers. PBMs run prescription drug benefit management programs on behalf of insurers and sometimes other payers, like Medicaid or Medicare Part D. PBMs negotiate drug prices with drug manufacturers and pharmacies. So they are middlemen in the drug distribution chain. They compose and maintain lists of drugs "covered" by the insurer (lists known as formularies). PBMs contract with pharmacies to reimburse for drugs dispensed. The least transparent link in this drug distribution chain is the one between the PBM and the drug manufacturer. PBMs use their market power to negotiated rebates and discounts from the manufacturers. These murky rebates and discounts are considered by some to be kick-backs.

PBMs are exempt from anti-kickback laws, so they may end up inflating the cost of prescription drugs. Here's the most succinct explanation of PBM kick-backs that I've found (12):

Pharmaceutical companies point the finger at pharmacy benefit managers who work for the insurers.

Each insurer has a list that shows which drugs it will pay for and in what order. Pharma companies want to be at the top of the list, so they pay rebates to PBMs to ensure good placements. The money is split with the insurers.

Still confused? Don't give up yet.

Here's an example. In 2019 the drug company Eli Lilly marketed a half-price version of its insulin drug, Humalog, to make this life-saving drug more affordable. Another company, Gilead, formed a subsidiary to produce "authorized generics" of its two revolutionary hepatitis C treatments, Harvoni and Epclusa, at prices more than 70% lower than the brand-name drugs. In 2018, Amgen and Sanofi introduced less costly versions of their cholesterol-lowering drugs (for patients unresponsive to standard statins) at 60% below the original prices. According to an opinion piece in *The Washington Times* (46):

> ...the system is not working: These less expensive versions of innovative drugs are not available to many seniors because of how insurance companies and their negotiators (known as "pharmacy benefit managers" or PBMs) design drug coverage via formularies, particularly in Medicare. A perfect case study is cardiovascular disease, the No. 1 cause of death in the United States: For the past 14 months, in many instances, United Healthcare formulary design kept patients on the more expensive versions of the Sanofi and Amgen cholesterol medicines which came coupled with a high out-of-pocket co-insurance for the patient. Further, CVS (which is merging with insurance company Aetna) admitted to creating barriers for patients by requiring doctors to provide a "documented

clinical reason" for prescribing the identical, cheaper version of the same medicine. Today in Medicare, CVS continues to block affordable access to the lower cost versions by not covering these medicines anywhere on their national formulary, effectively dissuading a patient at high risk for a heart attack or stroke from purchasing the medicine prescribed by his/her cardiologist.

Why would insurance companies and PBMs want to keep paying for the more expensive version of an identical drug? The answer lies in the backward way drugs are priced in America. Drug manufacturers set the "list price" of a drug the same way a car dealership lists the price of cars or colleges list the price of tuition. What's actually paid by an insurer in the final transaction is usually steeply discounted from the starting price by the drug company "rebating" a portion — 40 percent on average, oftentimes more — to the PBM/insurance company (which then pocket it). That negotiation should result in reduced out-of-pocket drug costs for seniors. The problem is that this model results in perverse incentives.

From *Forbes* magazine in 2019 (60):

All major health insurers now operate PBMs. UnitedHealth Group, owns the OptumRx PBM; Anthem is rolling out its new IngenioRx PBM; CVS Health, which owns the Caremark PBM, bought health insurance giant Aetna last year; and Humana has for years owned and operated its own PBM.

In 2017, Henry Waxman and associates produced a report (10) detailing many of the reasons for high drug prices, along with possible solutions. Here are a few of the causes they cited (direct quotes):

- Some manufacturers create, or take advantage of, natural monopolies for drugs [via patents] that enable them to significantly increase prices.
- The lack of robust competition among manufacturers of generic drugs results in less price competition and higher prices.
- The lack of price competition among biologics and biosimilars results in higher prices.
- Anticompetitive behavior by some manufacturers undermines competition, resulting in higher prices.
- Some manufacturers use current patent-protection policies for brand-name drugs to extend monopoly pricing.
- The pharmaceutical distribution system does not make essential pricing information available to patients, providers, and payers at the point of care — information that patients and their providers need when deciding on the best course of treatment.
- Federal law imposes limitations on state authority to negotiate prices for Medicaid and implement other price-related measures to reduce high drug prices.

Federal law prevented Medicare from negotiating drug prices for the benefit of Part D enrollees until very recently. Legislation passed in 2022 is allowing Medicare to negotiate prices for 10 drugs, with "maximum fair prices" to be set in 2024 and negotiated prices to take effect in 2026 (92). More drugs are expected to be added in coming years. Medicare expects to save nearly $100 billion over 10 years. Naturally, the drug industry has filed lawsuits to halt the process.

9. EXCESSIVE REGULATION

Without a doubt, a degree of governmental regulation of healthcare is necessary and good for the public. For example, it's a good idea to be sure that drugs are safe and effective before they are brought to market. It's beneficial to ensure that medical doctors are well-trained before they get licensed, and I applaud state medical boards that discipline unethical and harmful physicians, de-licensing them if necessary.

But regulations always carry a cost that is hidden and often difficult to calculate. That cost will be paid through higher prices, higher taxes, reduced wages or job opportunities, or fewer available services and products. Sometimes the benefits of the regulations are worth the cost.

On the other hand, poorly designed regulations clearly cause more harm than good. They can strangle innovation, impede job creation, and stifle economic growth. They waste resources and erode confidence in our government. In short, they harm the folks they are supposed to help. Always be on guard when you hear, "I'm from the government and I'm here to help you."

Hospitals, health systems, and post-acute care providers must comply with 629 discrete regulatory requirements from CMS (Centers for Medicare and Medicaid Services), Office of Inspector General, Office for Civil Rights, and Office of the National Coordinator for Health Information Technology. This is according to the American Hospital Association (14). The regulated facilities spend $39 billion on administrative activities related to regulatory compliance. This doesn't even include state-level regulatory requirements. Sixty-three percent of the $39 billion goes to documenting 1) hospital "conditions of participation" adherence, and 2) billing/coverage verification processes. The average-sized community hospital (161 beds) employs 59 full-time equivalents to maintain compliance.

Here's a specific example of federal regulation of healthcare. Since 2014, in order to maintain their existing Medicare and Medicaid reimbursement levels, all public and private healthcare providers have been required to adopt electronic health records (EHRs). Providers not in compliance with meaningful use of EHRs are penalized with lower reimbursement rates. These medical record systems are not cheap. Patients are paying for them via higher patient care fees and insurance premiums. Do you really need the federal government in the exam room when you go to the doctor for your eczema? Why not let expert medical providers decide if an EHR is necessary or not?

Here are a few of the federal laws that require regulatory compliance by various healthcare entities:

HIPAA - Health Insurance Portability and Accountability Act of 1996

PSQIA – Patient Safety and Quality Improvement Act of 2005

HITECH – Health Information Technology and Clinical Health Act of 2009

HRRP – Hospital Readmissions Reduction Program in

2010

MACRA – Medicare Access & CHIP Reauthorization Act of 2015

Of course, the government (or its contractors) employ a legion of bureaucrats to monitor and ensure compliance by healthcare providers. And you can bet the regulations are changed periodically to keep folks on their toes. Fines and other punishments for failure to comply can be quite stiff. For example, fines for running afoul of HIPAA (Health Insurance Portability and Accountability Act) can be up to $50,000 per violation.

10. DEFENSIVE MEDICINE

"Defensive medicine" typically refers to physicians ordering tests or consultations to minimize their risk of getting sued in the event of an adverse patient outcome. For instance, if you see primary care physician Dr. Singh regarding a headache, she can diagnose you accurately nine out of 10 times based on physical exam and your description of the headache. She could tell you, "I'm pretty sure you have a sinus headache. Let's treat it with an antihistamine and decongestant nasal spray, and I bet it'll go away. If not, we'll consider other possibilities." Or Dr. Singh could think to herself, "This is a sinus headache," but tell you, "I'm not entirely sure what's causing your headache. Let's get a brain MRI scan and consult a neurologist." This latter course is defensive medicine. The cost of care just rose by an order of magnitude, but at least Dr Singh's liability is reduced and it didn't cost her anything. The MRI scan has perhaps a one in a thousand chance of altering headache management. Oh, and if you went to the emergency department instead of the clinic, you'd get a head CT scan, regardless of your story, maybe before you ever saw the doctor. You just spent $4,000 on your sinus headache.

It's hard to estimate the cost of defensive medicine, but it's a real thing. Consider this 2014 article in *JAMA Internal Medicine* (20):

> In this study of hospital medicine services at 3 institutions in a health system, 28% of [physician] orders and 13% of costs were judged to be at least partially defensive, but only 2.9% of costs were completely defensive. Most costs were due to potentially unnecessary hospitalization. Defensive medicine practices varied substantially, but physicians who wrote the most defensive orders spent less than those who wrote fewer such orders, highlighting the disconnect between physician beliefs about defensive medicine and their contribution to costs.

> In 2008, Massachusetts internists reported that 27% of CT scans, 16% of laboratory tests and 14% of hospital admissions were ordered due to concerns about liability. We allowed our physicians to offer a graded response, which revealed that defensiveness is not absolute. Compared to the previous study, our respondents reported higher percentages of defensive medicine, but lower percentages of completely defensive medicine (2% of radiology, 6% of laboratory testing and 2% of hospital days).

Thomas Sullivan writing in 2018 at *Policy & Health* (21) suggests that 2.4% of U.S. healthcare spending is due to defensive medicine:

The study, conducted by authors from Harvard University and the University of Melbourne, estimated that defensive medicine is costing America $45.6 billion annually (in 2008 dollars), accounting for more than 80% of the $55.6 billion total yearly cost of the medical liability system. And this number did not "attempt to estimate social costs or benefits of the malpractice system, such as damage to physicians' reputations or any deterrent effect it may provide."

According to Michelle Mello, one of the study authors and a professor of law and public health at the Harvard School of Public Health, the study include (sic) estimates of defensive medicine costs both for hospitals ($38.8 billion) and for physicians ($6.8 billion). These estimates were calculated by looking at costs in high- and low-liability environments, and the authors reasoned "that the difference represents spending due to fear of being sued — i.e. defensive medicine."

Nearly all physicians are required to have "malpractice insurance," also known as professional liability insurance. The cost of medical malpractice insurance varies widely from state to state and by specialty. To get you in the ballpark, primary care physicians average $12,000/year for insurance, specialists ~$21,000. OB-GYN and specialty surgeons pay the most for insurance, which could approach $100,000 or more per year. The insurance pays for legal defense of malpractice allegations, and for lawsuit settlements and court judgments. Liability insurance premiums are an overhead cost of doing business. The cost is ultimately paid by the consumer.

But there's more to consider than the insurance premiums and defensive medicine costs. Lawsuits take an emotional toll, especially a doctor's first lawsuit, and they steal physician time away from patient care. Once sued, a physician tends to practice even more defensive medicine.

Overall, changes in the practice of defensive medicine and in malpractice litigation, i.e., tort reform, seem unlikely to have a major effect on cost of medical care.

11. INSURANCE MANDATES

I introduced you to this concept with a paragraph in the "third-party interference" section above. It's important enough to warrant its own section.

Health insurers are regulated primarily by the 50 states and secondarily by the federal government. Among the various states, there are over 1,900 mandates for specific benefits and coverage. For instance, states can mandate coverage for services from acupuncturists and naturopaths even though most physicians don't consider those approaches science-based. Additionally, 2010's Patient Protection and Affordable Care Act (aka ACA or Obamacare) requires that insurances on the "Exchanges" and in the small group and individual markets provide for 10 Essential Health Benefits (EHBs). These mandates include maternity and newborn care and pediatric services even if you're 55-years-old and your family is complete. Obamacare also mandates breastfeeding equipment and supplies, birth control, plus mental health and substance abuse services. CMS made changes to the original mandates in 2019, ostensibly giving individual states more flexibility in formulating coverage requirements. See "State Insurance Mandates and the ACA Essential Benefits Provisions" for a few of the mind-numbing details (22).

The ACA instituted two very popular requirements for Obamacare-compliant plans. It prevents insurance companies from cancelling insurance just because you get sick and start costing them money. And it prevents insurers from charging higher premiums for pre-existing conditions. Despite my research into healthcare reform, I don't know if these protections apply to *all* insurance plans.

Maybe you're willing to pay out of pocket for routine physicals, screening lab work, sore throats, bronchitis, minor rashes, and basic x-rays. Maybe you're happy with the sex you were born with and don't want insurance coverage for a sex-change operation. Maybe you're 55-years-old and have never had mental health problems or drug abuse issues. What if you want health insurance that covers only expensive major medical problems, like invasive cancer, heart attacks, strokes, major trauma, and hospitalizations? Well, your state insurance commissioner may not allow that due to the aforementioned mandates. The commissioner thinks he knows better than you what you need and is backed up by the force of law. So you or your employer end up paying for coverage that you'll never use. You're paying for maternity and pediatric care yet never had fun making the baby.

12. LOW OR NO INSURANCE DEDUCTIBLES

Ever heard the phrase, "skin in the game"? If you have skin in the game, it means you personally have something tangible to gain or lose depending on the outcome of a decision or course of action. Nassim Nicholas Taleb wrote a book about that in 2018, called *Skin In the Game: Hidden Asymmetries In Daily Life*. Taleb's book thesis is that skin in the game is necessary for fairness, commercial efficiency, and risk management, as well as being necessary to understand the world. Taleb is right.

In the arena of healthcare, "skin in the game" would figuratively refer to having a personal cost to pay for various healthcare and insurance decisions. Do you have skin in the game when your employer or the government chooses your health insurance plan? Do you have skin in the game when your health insurer tells you which provider you'll see, which hospital you'll use? Well, you do, literally. But not figuratively.

A substantial but diminishing fraction of Americans have very rich and comprehensive insurance coverage with very little financial outlay needed from the consumer, once premiums are paid. Need an office visit? $20 out-of-pocket. Need an ED visit? $100 max from the consumer. These lucky folks don't have much financial skin in the game. They don't bat an eye when their doctor after an initial visit for dizziness recommends a neurology consultation, cardiology consultation, brain MRI, EKG, echocardiogram, and lab work. No skin in the game. The charges are up to $10,000 now, but insurance is paying for it. You could argue that this medical care isn't too expensive: it's too cheap. The consumer is only paying $20 for the physician office visits.

But increasing numbers of consumers (four in 10) now find themselves in high-deductible health plans, with deductibles ranging from perhaps $1,000 to $5,000 or even higher. Remember that health insurance doesn't start paying part of the bill until the yearly deductible is met. $5,000 is definitely skin in the game range. And $1,000 is too, for many of us. A Federal Reserve survey (108) in 2022 found that 37% of Americans would struggle to come up with even $400 for an unexpected expense, like a car repair. They're living paycheck to paycheck. Nearly one in five said the most they could cover using only their savings was under $100.

A fortuitous side effect of these high insurance deductibles is that more consumers are shopping for their healthcare like they shop for every other consumer good or service. Consumers are demanding to know prices for drugs, office visits, diagnostic studies, and newborn baby delivery. Just like prices for LASIK eye surgery, cosmetic surgery, and over-the-counter drugs are routinely available. By the way, have you noticed that over-the-counter drugs and LASIK and cosmetic surgery are NOT covered by health insurance, so you don't have that third-party interference and middle men that need to be paid? This high-deductible situation is one of the reasons that the rate of healthcare cost inflation has moderated in the last few years. Unfortunately, high deductibles may also dissuade folks from getting necessary healthcare.

13. GOVERNMENT ESSENTIALLY MANDATES EMERGENCY DEPARTMENT CARE REGARDLESS

OF ABILITY TO PAY

Imagine that you own a successful restaurant. You started it with a $150,000 loan. For the first two years of operation you couldn't take a paycheck for yourself – despite 80-hour work weeks - because there was no money left after paying employees, rent, utilities, payroll taxes, loan payments, etc. Now in your third year, you can start paying yourself. Word of mouth has gotten around and you're busier than ever. Customers are so satisfied that you can even raise your prices a bit. The future's so bright, you gotta wear shades.

But then the federal government this year passes unfunded legislation mandating that you must feed everyone who shows up hungry at your door, for free if they have no ability to pay. You have one loophole: you don't have to feed them if you can prove they're not hungry. Welcome to your new normal: the Emergency Meal, Table, and Libation Act (EMTALA) of 2024. Your restaurant will always be crowded, with long waits for tables, folks who used to eat at home are coming in because it's convenient, your staff are surly because they're overworked, quality of food goes down because you can't afford the better ingredients, your expenses skyrocket while your revenue suffers despite higher menu prices, your old loyal customers complain because they remember the good old days, and you have to beg for donations and have bi-annual fundraisers like PBS. Oh, and you may not be able to take your salary this year.

This legislation is what the feds laid on hospital Emergency Departments in 1986. Only it wasn't about food, but about healthcare. Here are basic requirements of the Emergency Medical Treatment and Active Labor

Act (EMTALA) from a 2010 *AMA Journal of Ethics* article (23):

> To comply with the provisions of the act, any hospital that receives Medicare dollars must: (a) screen all patients who come to the ED to determine whether a medical emergency exists, (b) stabilize patients who have emergent conditions, and (c) restrict transfer of nonstabilized patients to cases in which a physician certifies that the benefits of the transfer outweigh the risks or the patient (or surrogate) requests a transfer in writing after knowing the risks involved.
>
> "Medical emergency" is broadly defined as the presence of symptoms of such severity that the absence of immediate medical attention could place the individual's health in jeopardy or result in serious impairment of bodily organs or function. In the case of pregnant women who are having contractions, a medical emergency exists when there is inadequate time for transfer before delivery or when transfer might threaten the health or safety of the woman or the unborn child.

Prior to EMTALA, public "charity" hospitals provided much of the emergency care to the indigent and Medicaid patients. Private hospitals provided some charity care, partly by cost-shifting: charging insured patients more than they otherwise would. (Is it really charity if you're using other peoples' money?) With the rise of managed care, this cost shifting may have dwindled. On the other hand, if you are un-insured or out-of-network, the hospital may sock it to ya, baby, billing for multiples of what they charge the insured patients.

A physician who violates EMTALA faces a fine of up to $50,000 for each violation. Hospitals are fined up to $104,826 per violation ($52,414 if hospital has under 100 beds). EMTALA has turned EDs-very expensive places-into the medical safety net for everyone in the U.S.

The American Hospital Association calculated that hospitals provided $43 billion in uncompensated care in 2020 (24). It's unclear what fraction of that was for free emergency department services. Emergency physicians and ED on-call physicians also "donate" their time to EMTALA patients. That must be worth hundreds of millions of dollars per year.

We don't force grocers to give away free food to those in need. Instead, we have the food stamp program - SNAP or Supplemental Nutrition Assistance Program – to provide food for the indigent. The cost is borne by the general population. We also have charity food banks, often operated by volunteers and funded by voluntary donations. On the other hand, the financial burden of EMTALA falls directly on hospitals and physicians. Of course, those costs in part must be passed on to the more well-off patients. Otherwise the provider goes out of business.

No physician or hospital administrator wants to throw indigent patients out in the cold to die alone and in misery. We just want a fair mechanism for financing their care.

14. PROVIDERS ARE INCENTIVIZED TO PROVIDE SERVICES

Sometimes in medicine, it's better to do *nothing* than to do *something*. Determining the best course takes dedicated time. But if you're paid very well to do something, and very little to do nothing, would that influence your decision-making?

Imagine a healthcare system in which providers are paid not for taking care of sickness but paid to keep people healthy in the first place. Paid to prevent disease and sickness. Paid for prolonging quality years of life. Well, that's not descriptive of much of the U.S. healthcare system. Perhaps the closest we come is a health maintenance organization which is given a pot of money yearly (insurance premiums) to keep a specified population healthy and pay for the inevitable illnesses that will arise. The HMO consists of care providers, hospitals, and diagnostic facilities that work as a team to keep the population as healthy as possible. Healthier folks use a lot less medical resources, right? So it should be a less expensive system. How do you keep the population healthier and out of the expensive sick-care portion of the HMO? It might look like this: 1) reasonable immunizations, 2) periodic physical exams with basic lab work, 3) science-based screening for cancer, heart disease, diabetes, hypertension, and cerebrovascular disease, 4) periodic screening for drug abuse and mental illness, 5) strong efforts to avoid obesity and promote exercise, 6) financial incentives for enrollees who demonstrate healthy behaviors, 7) financial bonuses for providers with higher compliance with preventive care guidelines, and 8) enforcement of science-based guidelines that prevent care providers from ordering unnecessary tests or procedures. Such a system might actually work to keep people heathier at lower overall cost. (That's debatable on another day.)

One major problem with it, however, is that the health benefits and financial savings typically aren't realized until at least 10-15 years later. By then, the consumer has long since moved on to a different job with a different health insurer. The HMO who invested in preventive care has helped their competitor, another insurance company. That's one reason why you don't often see a serious push for preventive medicine in the U.S.

Physicians are primarily trained to diagnose and treat sickness. Yes, they know prevention is also important and have training in that, too. But your typical physician in most settings is paid to diagnose and treat illness all day. The more patients she sees and treats, the more she's paid. And procedures are much more lucrative than cognitive services. "Cognitive" refers to obtaining a thorough history, doing a good physical exam, analyzing data, talking to the patient, etc. To maximize her pay, a physician is incentivized to see more patients and do more procedures. Unfortunately, too many physicians are seeing more patients than they can safely handle, and doing procedures that may not be medically necessary. That tends to drive up healthcare costs. Sometimes a physician may know it's wrong, but a supervisor is cracking the whip. Employed physicians at multi-physician clinics are tracked in terms of productivity. If Dr. Aggarwal is seeing 20% fewer patients per day than the average doc, he's going to be called to the principal's office. "You need to up your game, or else...." Doctors have bills to pay like everyone else. Have you ever been in a clinic that treats people like cattle? Do you think workers at a slaughterhouse talk to the cows?

Surgeon Atul Gawande wrote about such perverse incentives in 2015 (29):

> The one thing the medical profession is not rewarded for is providing better, higher-value care. We are financially rewarded either for doing more stuff or for securing monopoly power. In a fee-for-service payment system—a system of paying doctors and hospitals by pill and procedure—we are actually penalized for making the effort to organize and deliver care with the best service, quality, and efficiency we can.

15. GREED

Greed is an excessive and selfish desire for more of something (especially wealth, food, or power) than is deserved (or needed?). "Selfish" is a key component here. Selfish people are primarily concerned with their personal profit or pleasure, discounting or ignoring the consideration of others. You know greed is common.

All of us have the potential to be greedy. Including hospital administrators, politicians, physicians, insurance company executives, pharmaceutical executives, lawyers, clinic managers and support staff, etc.

But greed is not necessarily the same as wanting to maximize your legitimate income. The average NFL (National Football League) player was paid $2.8 million a year in 2023 (25). Is that more than they need or deserve? The average Major League Baseball player earned $4.9 million a year. Is that more than they need or deserve?

The average NBA (National Basketball Association) player earned $9.4 million a year. Is that more than they need or deserve? If you want those player's jobs and salaries, you can work for it and apply. Those guys aren't selfish. They're not discounting or ignoring the consideration of others. They bring their fans a lot of pleasure. They are simply earning what the market will bear.

Average hospitalist compensation was $319,000 in 2022 (93). As a hospitalist, I save lives on a regular basis. I'm paid well for it and I'm satisfied with my salary. Yet I don't make nearly as much as those professional sportsball players who are merely entertainers. I'm not bitter or jealous about it. I'm happy for them. The employment market determines what I'm worth financially. Like all healthy young folks, I could have taken a crack at professional sports when I was young, but never even tried.

A 2019 article at *Forbes* listed the 2018 salaries of the top earners (whether CEO or president) at the 82 largest non-profit hospitals in the U.S. (26). These hospitals are organized as *charities* under IRS code 501(c)(3). In 13 of the organizations, the top earner was paid between $5 and 21.6 million. In 61 organizations the top earner was paid between $1 and 5 million. In eight organizations, the pay was under $1 million. In my neck of the woods, Banner Health paid its president $34 million and executive vice president $12.4 million. Mind you, this is at a time when a **hypothetical American family of four covered by an average employer-sponsored preferred provider organization (PPO)** is paying $28,000 a year for healthcare. **That $28,000 includes more than $12,000 in premiums and out-of-pocket charges plus reduced** pay and other forms of worker compensation to cover ever-growing health care costs (32). Are those CEO salaries more than the executives need or deserve? If you want those salaries, get the necessary education and apply for the job.

It doesn't matter whether you're a cashier at Walmart or a trial lawyer in a downtown skyscraper, you naturally want to maximize your paycheck. That's not greed. It's self-interest. If Safeway is paying cashiers more, quit and get a job there. If you want a doctor's paycheck, go to medical school. The employment market ultimately determines your pay, with some wiggle room depending on your personality, connections, and a few other factors. If you are the only neurosurgeon in a town of 250,000, you have the potential to be very richly rewarded. Neurosurgeons are among the highest paid physicians, averaging about $550,000 per year. If you want that job, go for it.

Greed is an excessive and selfish desire for more of something than is deserved (or needed?). "Selfish" is a key component here. If you're paying the $20,000 a month nursing home bill for your aged and disabled mother, you need a higher salary than otherwise. That doesn't make you greedy.

I'm not sure how to counteract greed. We can endlessly debate how much income is "needed." The only countervailing force may be an open, transparent, free market. When your local "charity" hospital has its annual fund-raising drive, will your donation be as generous when you know the CEO is making $10 million a year?

Some physicians are greedy, too. See #14. Believe it or

not, even politicians and government bureaucrats can be greedy.

16. UN-ENFORCED ANTI-TRUST AND CONSUMER PROTECTION LAWS. MONOPOLIES

I can't say it any better than the Federal Trade Commission (35): "Free and open markets are the foundation of a vibrant economy. Aggressive competition among sellers in an open marketplace gives consumers — both individuals and businesses — the benefits of lower prices, higher quality products and services, more choices, and greater innovation. The FTC's competition mission is to enforce the rules of the competitive marketplace — the antitrust laws. These laws promote vigorous competition and protect consumers from anticompetitive mergers and business practices."

Think about all of the advancements in telecommunications, computers, automobiles, manufacturing, and agriculture over the last half-century. We have better products at lower prices. That's because of competition, innovation, and technology. There's no reason that formula won't work for healthcare. When rewarded, competition leads to innovation and new/improved technology. Monopolies are anti-competitive by definition.

Have you noticed hospital mergers in your area? It's a national trend, but is it good for patients? No, according to a 2020 article at *New England Journal of Medicine* (27):

> The hospital industry has consolidated substantially during the past two decades and at an accelerated pace since 2010. Multiple studies have shown that hospital

mergers have led to higher prices for commercially insured patients, but research about effects on quality of care is limited.

According to this study:

Hospital acquisition by another hospital or hospital system was associated with modestly worse patient experiences and no significant changes in readmission or mortality rates.

Large hospital systems are powerful political entities. For example, they are the largest employers in 16 states (28). Politicians are hesitant to make enemies of them by going against their wishes. Drive through any U.S. town of 20,000 to 50,000 population; the most modern building and largest employer is likely to be a hospital.

Surgeon and public-health researcher Atul Gawande wrote at *The New Yorker* (29):

When your grocery store is the only one in town, it can jack up prices without losing customers. The same goes for hospitals. The study found that hospital prices in monopoly markets are fifteen per cent higher than in those with four or more hospitals.

Christopher Jacobs wrote at *The Federalist* in 2018 (30):

Hospitals responded to the law [Obamacare or PPACA] by buying up other hospitals, increasing market share in an attempt to gain more negotiating "clout" against health insurers. That leverage allows them to demand clauses such as those preventing price transparency, or preventing insurers from developing smaller networks that only include efficient or better-quality providers.

In addition to merging and consolidating amongst themselves, hospitals have also gone on a buying spree for physician practices, acting again to obtain larger market share, and have a "one-stop-shop" for health care services. The *[Wall Street] Journal* cites University of California data showing that, since Obamacare's passage, the percentage of doctors employed by hospitals rose from 27.7 percent in 2010 to 43.5 percent in 2016. As a result, a plurality of American physicians now work for hospitals, rather than in medical groups or independent practice.

Here again, industry consolidation begets higher prices. In many cases, hospitals can charge more for services provided by an "outpatient facility" as opposed to one provided by a "doctor's office." In some circumstances, the patient will receive the same service, provided by the same doctor, in the same office, but will end up getting charged a higher price—merely because, by buying the physician practice, the hospital can reclassify the office and procedure as taking place in an "outpatient facility."

The next few pages deep-dive into the monopoly issue. Fair warning: It's esoteric and boring to most readers! It's for healthcare policy wonks only. Feel free to jump ahead to the next cause of high-cost healthcare: #17 Over-utilization of specialist care instead of primary care.

In a scholarly article at *Oregon Law Review* and published in 2011, attorneys Clark Havighurst and Barak Richman wrote (31):

At the same time that health insurance ameliorates monopoly's usual adverse effects on output and allocative efficiency, it greatly exacerbates monopoly's other objectionable effect, the redistribution of wealth from consumers to powerful firms. In the textbook model, the monopolist's higher price enables it to capture for itself much of the welfare gain, or "surplus," that consumers would have enjoyed if they had been able to purchase the valued good or service at a low, competitive price. In health care, insurance puts the monopolist in an even stronger position by greatly weakening the constraint on its pricing freedom ordinarily imposed by the limits of consumers' willingness or ability to pay. This effect appears in theory as a steepening of the demand curve for the monopolized good or service. The extraordinary profits that health insurance makes available to powerful sellers are earned mostly at the expense not of direct purchasers—insurers or patients—but of consumers bearing the cost of insurance.

* * *

Thus, many factors besides certain judges' sanguine attitude toward nonprofit [hospital] monopolies contributed to what should now appear—once one recognizes the extraordinary pricing freedom that U.S.-style health insurance confers on monopolist providers and suppliers—to have been a colossally important failure of antitrust enforcement. Today, in large part because of hospital mergers and other consolidations, there are few markets in which price competition keeps prices for specific hospital and other health care services and goods near their marginal cost.

* * *

A first order of business in fighting provider market power is to prevent accountable care organizations (ACOs) from aggregating such power. The PPACA encourages providers to integrate themselves in ACOs for the purpose of implementing "best practices" and thereby providing coordinated care of good quality at low cost. As an inducement for providers to form and practice within these presumptively more efficient entities, the PPACA instructs the Medicare program to share with an ACO any cost savings it can demonstrate. Observers are now expressing concern, however, that ACOs—whatever their value to Medicare may be—will attain and exercise substantial market power vis-à-vis private health plans. *The New York Times* has reported "a growing frenzy of mergers involving hospitals, clinics and doctor groups eager to share costs and savings, and cash in on the [ACO program's] incentives." In fact, providers' main purpose in forming ACOs may not be to achieve cost savings to be shared with Medicare but to strengthen their market power over purchasers in the private sector.

Although the PPACA appears designed to achieve the benefits of vertical integration for Medicare and its beneficiaries, it inevitably invites horizontal integration that creates new market power in private markets. The formation of ACOs should therefore be subject to close antitrust scrutiny.

* * *

In conclusion:

Our principal point is that health insurance, especially as it is designed and administered in the United States, hugely expands monopolists' pricing freedom, making monopoly's wealth-redistributing and misallocative effects substantially more serious than monopoly's effects usually are. Although this point has been almost completely absent from the antitrust and economics literature, its importance would seem to dwarf all other considerations in accounting for the extraordinarily high cost of U.S. health care.

To mitigate the harms from provider market power, we advise vigorous, rather than tentative or circumspect, enforcement of the antitrust laws.

* * *

Unfortunately, health insurers are far less eager to contest provider market power and to act as aggressive purchasing agents of consumers than they would be if consumers were both aware of the true cost of their health coverage and conscious that they, rather than someone else [e.g., employers], are paying for it.

Currently, when it comes to their health care, insured consumers are unduly reluctant to accept anything less than the very best. U.S. health plans are therefore inadequately incentivized to reduce costs and overly hesitant to adopt innovative strategies with associated legal or political risks.

Open Market has an article on hospitals and monopolies (33):

What explains these disparities [between the U.S. and other OECD countries]? One large and often overlooked factor is the increasing monopolization of health care markets. The trend includes growing market concentration in pharmaceuticals, medical devices, and health insurance. Yet even more consequential for the cost of health care is the increasing monopolization found among hospitals, which accounts for the majority of U.S. health care spending.

Not a single highly competitive hospital market

remains in any region of the United States, according to the standard metric used by the Federal Trade Commission to measure degrees of concentration, the Herfindahl-Hirschman Index (HHI). By the same measure, the hospital markets in 90% of Metropolitan Statistical Areas are officially highly concentrated.

When hospitals buy out their competitors, the effect is almost always higher prices. According to a literature survey by the Robert Wood Johnson Foundation, "The magnitude of price increases when hospitals merge in concentrated markets is typically quite large, most exceeding 20 percent." A recent and widely discussed study by Yale economist Zack Cooper and others has found that if you stay in a hospital that faces no competition, your bill will be $1,900 higher on average than if you stay in a hospital facing four or more competitors. If hospital mergers are creating efficiency gains, it's hard to find instances in which the savings are being shared with customers. Even among hospitals operating in different regions, when mergers occur, the effect is higher prices, typically running between 7 percent and 17 percent, according to studies.

The article states that the FTC (Federal Trade Commission) is not allowed to prosecute anti-competitive practices of non-profit organizations, which are nearly half of all hospitals in the U.S.

The *Open Markets* report continues:

Hospitals have cited the theory that their integration [mergers] will lead to economies of scale that will reduce health care inflation and allow for better-integrated care. Yet in the absence of coherent policies for preserving and managing competition in health care markets, the real-world results of health care consolidation, aside from many more closed hospitals, has mostly been price gouging and increasingly acute price discrimination against those who lack the market power to stand up to monopolistic providers.

Going forward, the local monopolies that now dominate health care delivery present a deep threat to meaningful health care reform. Even under a "single-payer" or "Medicare for all" payer system, health care monopolies might well have a power akin to sole-source Pentagon contractors as their size, political power, and lack of competition allows them to set their own prices. Meaningful reform of the American health care system requires shrewd use of competition policy to tame monopolies and restructure health care markets.

So it appears that monopolies are contributing to the high cost of healthcare in the U.S. The primary antitrust laws are the Sherman Act of 1890, The Federal Trade Commission Act of 1914, and the Clayton Act of 1914. From the FTC (34):

The antitrust laws proscribe unlawful mergers and business practices in general terms, leaving courts to decide which ones are illegal based on the facts of each case. Courts have applied the antitrust laws to changing markets, from a time of horse and buggies to the present digital age. Yet for over 100 years, the antitrust laws have had the same basic objective: to protect the process of competition for the benefit of consumers, making sure there are strong incentives for businesses to operate efficiently, keep prices down, and keep quality up.

The key word in that paragraph is competition. The Sherman Act outlaws "every contract, combination, or conspiracy in [unreasonable] restraint of trade," and any "monopolization, attempted monopolization, or conspiracy or combination to monopolize." Flagrant examples include arrangements among competing individuals or businesses to fix prices, divide markets, or rig bids. Violations may be prosecuted by the Department of Justice, and the will to enforce the Act varies over time and according to which political party is in power.

The Federal Trade Commission Act bans "unfair methods of competition" and "unfair or deceptive acts or practices." Since all violations of the Sherman Act also violate the FTC Act, it can bring cases under the FTC Act against the same kinds of activities that violate the Sherman Act.

Directly from the FTC website: The Clayton Act addresses specific practices that the Sherman Act does not clearly prohibit, such as mergers and interlocking directorates (that is, the same person making business decisions for competing companies). Section 7 of the Clayton Act prohibits mergers and acquisitions where the effect "may be substantially to lessen competition, or to tend to create a monopoly." As amended by the Robinson-Patman Act of 1936, the Clayton Act also bans certain discriminatory prices, services, and allowances in dealings between merchants. The Clayton Act was amended again in 1976 by the Hart-Scott-Rodino Antitrust Improvements

Act to require companies planning large mergers or acquisitions to notify the government of their plans in advance.

The Clayton Act was amended by the Robinson-Patman Act of 1936 (36):

> A seller charging competing buyers different prices for the same "commodity" or discriminating in the provision of "allowances" — compensation for advertising and other services — may be violating the Robinson-Patman Act. This kind of price discrimination may give favored customers an edge in the market that has nothing to do with their superior efficiency. Price discriminations are generally lawful, particularly if they reflect the different costs of dealing with different buyers or are the result of a seller's attempts to meet a competitor's offering.

Robinson-Patman may come into play in the area of pharmaceuticals: sales, discounts, pharmacy benefits management companies, pharmacies and insurance companies owning PBMs, generic versus brand-name drugs, etc.

Also note that most states have their own antitrust laws that can be enforced by state attorneys general (if there is political willingness) and private plaintiffs.

Some healthcare reform writers consider a drug patent, a program started in 1925, to be a monopoly. I disagree. If we want new and better drugs, we have to financially reward those who do the intellectual and physical work to develop them. Patent abuse and patent duration are worth a debate, but not here and now.

17. OVER-UTILIZATION OF SPECIALIST CARE INSTEAD OF PRIMARY CARE

Primary care providers are typically defined as family physicians, general internists, general pediatricians, and general practitioners. Plus the physician assistants and nurse practitioners that do similar work. (Some also consider ob-gyns to be primary care.) Primary care practice is characterized by:

- First contact with the healthcare system
- Longitudinality (following a patient over longer periods of time)
- Comprehensiveness
- Coordination of care with others in the health system
- Accessibility
- Personal or family-centeredness (as contrasted with specific disease or organ-centeredness)
- Community orientation
- More overall attention to prevention as compared to specialist care

A third of U.S. physicians work in primary care. Most other OECD countries have a significantly higher percentage of physicians in primary care. The proportion of U.S. physicians practicing primary care has been falling gradually for over a half century. The trend is driven by increasingly complex technology and the significantly higher pay, prestige, and respect given to specialists and subspecialists. Some specialists have a better lifestyle (e.g., fewer work hours, no night or weekend calls). The higher pay helps reduce medical school debt (75% of med school graduates have school debt, and it averages $200,000).

Leiyi Shi at Johns Hopkins Bloomberg School of Public Health (37) wrote in 2012 that:

> Studies conducted in industrialized countries, such as member nations of the Organization for Economic Cooperation and Development (OECD), do indicate that stronger primary care systems are generally associated with better population health outcomes including lower mortality rates, rates of premature death and hospitalizations for ambulatory care sensitive conditions, and higher infant birth weight, life expectancy, and satisfaction with the healthcare system. Studies in the USA have also indicated that greater primary care availability in a community is correlated with both better health outcomes and a decrease in utilization of more expensive types of health services, such as hospitalizations and emergency department (ED) visits.

We learned earlier that most OECD countries also have significantly less expensive healthcare systems than the U.S.

You'd think that having a predominance of specialists, with the high-technology available to them, would lead to lower death rates, right? Not according to this 2005 study at Health Affairs (38):

> Analyses at the county level show lower mortality rates where there are more primary care physicians, but this is not the case for specialist supply. These findings confirm those of previous studies at the state and

other levels. Increasing the supply of specialists will not improve the United States' position in population health relative to other industrialized countries, and it is likely to lead to greater disparities in health status and outcomes. Adverse effects from inappropriate or unnecessary specialist use may be responsible for the absence of relationship between specialist supply and mortality.

Our predominance of specialists drives up the cost of healthcare without improving population longevity.

Increasing the role of primary care providers by itself will not necessarily lower overall healthcare costs. Here are some reasons why. Remember that a plurality of physicians now work for hospital systems or other employed models. Many systems put undue pressure on PCPs to increase volume of patients seen. Physician pay may be partially based on volume seen. For instance, I have many years' experience as an office-based internist seeing a heavy Medicare workload. Medicare patient are 65 or older and often have multiple complicated medical problems. Not just a sore throat. Not just an ear ache. Not just poison ivy. They have hypertension, diabetes, arthritis, emphysema, and dizziness, all to be addressed at the same office visit. A good, ethical internist can only see a maximum of 18-20 of these patients in a day at the office. Employed physicians may be pressured to see 25-30 or more per day. Trust me, quality of care usually suffers. That employed physician may decide he needs her job, or the incentive bonus pay, and let that quality (and patient) suffer. This pressure to produce the volume is a major reason so many PCPs refer you out to a subspecialist to care for a problem that the PCP could handle if simply given the time. The subspecialist is happy to get the referral, and the PCP meets his production goal. The docs don't care, especially since they're not paying for it and don't have to endure the inconvenience. If excessive and expensive subspecialty care is the result, the insurance company simply raises insurance premiums. Talk about perverse incentives!

18. INSURANCE PAYS FOR TOO MUCH, INSTEAD OF ONLY CATASTROPHIC CARE

In the early days of health insurance, it only paid for very expensive, unforeseen problems, like major trauma, invasive cancer, and hospitalizations. This used to be called catastrophic coverage. Over time, insurance transmogrified into paying for relatively minor things (after a small deductible or co-pay), like poison ivy, lice infestation, tension headaches, insomnia, allergic rhinitis, toenail trimming, mole removal, constipation, transient diarrhea, vague dizziness, low back pain, and ingrown hairs. Insurance turned into first-dollar coverage, prepaid healthcare. Maybe the transition to covering everything was driven by higher prices. Or instead, maybe the higher charges were driven by the availability of insurance coverage.

Why isn't health insurance more like automobile or home insurance? Those insurance markets haven't become a major expense and problem for us like health insurance. You don't expect car insurance to pay for oil changes, gas, windshield wipers, and flat tires. If it did, you know the insurance would cost a lot more! Automobile insurance pays for major problems like a wreck that "totals" your car or pays for the damages to others in a wreck you're responsible for. You don't expect home insurance to pay for broken windows, leaky irrigation pipes, or a new roof every 20 years. You know the new roof will eventually need replacing so you save up for it. Your house burning down or demolished by a tornado is a catastrophe, and that's why you have insurance.

Unfortunately, federal and state regulations are making catastrophic health insurance plans fewer and far between. Whether for better or worse, the recent trend toward high deductibles, like $3,000 to $5,000, are turning health insurance into catastrophic plans. A deductible of $3,000 *is* a catastrophe for many individuals and families.

When healthcare is less expensive, catastrophic coverage is all you'll need. You'll be able to afford non-catastrophic care and pay out-of-pocket.

Oh, one more thing. Have you noticed that your employer doesn't arrange and pay for your auto and home insurance, and you don't lose the insurance when you change jobs? Why can't health insurance be the same?

19. WASTE, FRAUD, AND ABUSE (WFA)

Paraphrasing what Jesus said about the poor...waste, fraud, and abuse will always be with us. To some degree. Humans will be human. WFA accounts for perhaps 5 to 20% of healthcare costs. It's difficult to quantify. According to a 2020 article in the *American Journal of Public Health* (69), "estimates of waste varied from $600 billion to more than $1.9 trillion per year, or roughly $1800 to $5700 per person per year." The most interested parties in countering WFA should be the payers (insurance companies), regulators, and law enforcement. But how interested are they, really? All three can simply pass the WFA costs on to the consumer (patients, taxpayers, or whoever's paying the insurance premiums and deductibles), if they wish. So insurance companies, regulators (like CMS), and law enforcement should be weeding out waste, fraud, and abuse. What can you do as a consumer? If you're informed via an EOB (explanation of benefits) that someone did blood work, an office visit, and an MRI scan on you, but it never happened, tell your insurer. If you see WFA and can document it, tell someone in authority. I'm all in favor of pulling WFA out by the roots; that leaves more money for legitimate services or for reduction of insurance premiums or taxes. Remember, a 2.9% payroll tax goes to Medicare (39). In addition, thanks to Obamacare, employers are responsible for withholding an additional 0.9% Medicare Tax on an individual's wages paid in excess of $200,000 in a calendar year.)

IN SUMMARY

After review of all 19 issues above, we can condense them into six major issues (with significant overlap) to blame for the high cost of U.S. healthcare and that we should be able to do something about:

- Lack of price transparency
- Third-party interference in the patient-provider relationship (huge category)
- High administrative costs

- Unusually expensive drugs
- Monopolies & inadequate competition
- Successful lobbying by well-financed entities

I considered making "perverse incentives" one of the major issues, but it runs throughout all the top six.

CHAPTER 3: FOUNDATIONS OF HEALTHCARE REFORM

1. The heart of healthcare is the patient-provider relationship.

2. Healthcare must be science-based as much as possible, while recognizing that art is also a factor.

2. Relationships should be voluntary and mutually beneficial.

3. Patients (consumers) and providers (physician, nurses, hospitals, therapists, diagnostic facilities, pharmacies,

etc.) should have as much freedom as possible from third-party interference.

4. Core values that apply to consumers, providers, and support staff:

- the patient (consumer) is primary
- honesty
- trust
- simplicity
- transparency
- respect
- convenience
- benevolence
- collaboration
- reciprocity
- personal responsibility
- voluntary association
- freedom
- as a society, we take care of the needy when family isn't able

5. Charity is allowed and encouraged.

6. No one has to work for free. See the 13th amendment to U.S. Constitution (re: slavery). There is no right to healthcare since that would ultimately require forcing a provider to work for free.

7. Private-sector businesses cannot survive without profit.

8. If a healthcare provider makes a mistake that hurts a patient, the patient has a right to redress.

9. Regulations that simply make busywork for bureaucrats and healthcare providers should be

abolished.

10. Administrators, regulators, clerks, and others (even care providers) that are displaced by reform will find productive jobs elsewhere in the economy.

11. Foreign nationals in the U.S. who need healthcare will pay for it here or return to their own countries for care.

12. Successful reform will reduce healthcare costs to 5% of GDP instead of 17%. Prices for services will be sufficiently low that insurance "coverage" will not be necessary for most services and health conditions.

13. Technology, innovation, and competition will make healthcare less expensive, as it has in nearly all other areas of economic activity.

14. The U.S. Constitution is the supreme law of the land, so it should be honored.

15. We will reduce the burden on taxpayers.

16. We have better things to spend our money on than over-priced healthcare. Let citizens decide where to spend their money, not politicians, insurance companies, employers, and bureaucrats.

17. We recognize that if current trends continue (e.g., growth of government, aging sickly population, federal deficit spending), we are headed to a fiscal crisis.

18. Individuals and families have a responsibility to provide for the necessities of life, including medical care.

19. Healthcare is very important for all, therefore it is reasonable to subsidize health insurance with tax incentives.

Technology, innovation, and competition lower the cost of everything to which they're applied. There's no reason the formula won't work for healthcare. The engine driving the formula is financial reward. Successful technologists, innovators, and competitors must be allowed to profit.

Technology + innovation + competition + reward + time = minimal cost and maximal benefit

Now let's apply these foundational principles and create a new U.S. healthcare system.

CHAPTER 4:
SPECIFIC REFORMS
TO RESUSCITATE
U.S. HEALTHCARE

E arly-on in this book I mentioned 10 or so other high-income countries that spend significantly less on healthcare than the U.S. yet have better health outcomes. Why not just adopt one of their systems, some of which are characterized by heavier government planning and control? Some might call it socialized medicine, like the United Kingdom's National Health Service. Such a system is a serious consideration here and the percentage of the U.S population in favor is in the 40s.

BUT FIRST, WHAT ABOUT HEALTHCARE SYSTEMS IN OTHER COUNTRIES?

Don't worry, I'm not going to review all 195 countries. We'll look at ~15 countries, none of which I have personally visited other than the U.S. Reality on the ground may be very different than what I learned from the comfort of my office.

Let's start by defining the broad categories of healthcare system financing:

- **Private insurance**
- **Public insurance**: In some countries workers have social insurance, also called public insurance. Usually government withholds part of their wage (a payroll tax), which is divided between employee and employer. Additional funds may come from other taxes.
- **Single-payer healthcare**: One entity (public or quasi-public) collects funds and pays for healthcare on behalf of an entire population.
- **Out-of-pocket**

Many countries, like the U.S., are a blend of these financing mechanisms. For instance, In the U.S., our Veterans Health Administration is single-payer socialized medicine. Medicare is public single-payer insurance. Purely cosmetic surgical procedures and insurance deductibles are paid out-of-pocket. Employer-provided insurance is private insurance.

Universal Health Coverage (UHC) is often defined as

coverage for all members of a population for any kind of medical care, while not resulting in a significant immediate financial burden to individuals. UHC could be single-payer, public insurance, or social insurance. While "socialized medicine" is strictly integrated with the government, the government may or may not play a role in single-payer systems. In a socialized system, the government owns the buildings where care is rendered and it employs those who provide care. In a single-payer system, one entity pays for health care while hospitals, primary care clinics and other health care services are run by separate organizations, and doctors, nurses, and other health care providers are often employees of those organizations. "Single-payer" doesn't necessarily mean the government: the payer could be any insurance company that obtained the entirety of the health insurance market.

Other than the U.S., nearly all high-income countries provide Universal Health Coverage. So do Singapore, South Korea, and Malaysia, which I mention because they rank highly in several "best healthcare systems" lists. While the U.S. does not provide universal coverage, it covers 91% of the population.

Here's an over-simplified overview of healthcare financing systems in a few high-income countries and Malaysia (upper-middle-income):

- **Australia**: Single-payer, government-funded Medicare. Half of residents also buy subsidized supplementary insurance to pay for private hospital care and dental services.

- **Canada**: Single-payer, government-funded.

Canadian Medicare covers 70% of healthcare costs; private insurance pays for 30%. Supplemental insurance is carried by 70% of residents. Two-thirds of Canadians have private insurance to pay for prescription drugs, dental care, etc.

- **France**: Social insurance. Statutory health insurance is mandatory, funded by various taxes, including payroll taxes paid by employers and employees. Nearly all residents buy private voluntary supplemental insurance to help with co-pays, balance billing, dental and vision care, etc. Employers may help pay for it. Private insurance pays for ~13% of total healthcare expenditures.

- **Germany**: Public-private social insurance. About 88% of residents are enrolled in compulsory not-for-profit insurance provided by "sickness funds." Healthcare is funded for by payroll taxes shared equally by ensured employees and their employers. Germans above a certain income level can opt out of public insurance and buy private instead. Chancellor Otto von Bismarck's Health Insurance Act of 1883 established the world's first social health insurance system.

- **Japan**: Public insurance is mandatory (usually government withholds part of wage, divided between employee and employer). Citizens pay premiums and 30% co-insurance for most services. Sixty % of insurance is employment-based; the rest is "residence-based" (for the unemployed and/or elderly). The national government regulates nearly all aspects of the system. Health expenditures are funded by taxes (42%), mandatory individual contributions (42%), and out-of-pocket expenses (14%). Seventy % of residents have supplementary private insurance but it seems to function more as life or short-term disability insurance.

- **Netherlands**: Private insurance. Adults must purchase statutory insurance from nonprofit private insurers of their choosing. Otherwise they are fined. Children are automatically covered. Less than 1% of the population is uninsured. Healthcare is financed through payroll taxes paid by employers, general taxation, insurance premiums paid by individuals, and copayments. A large majority of the population also purchases voluntary supplemental insurance to help with expenses not paid by statutory insurance.

- **Malaysia**: Public-private mix, two-tiered. The public system, funded by taxes, provides universal access. Most residents use the public system for a nominal fee. There is also a large and thriving private system that caters to higher-income residents and medical travelers from other countries. In 2020, there were more private than government-owned hospitals. Most physicians speak English. Many doctors, especially specialists, gravitate to the private system, presumably for better working conditions, lower patient volumes, and/or higher pay. The private system is sustained by out-of-pocket payments and private insurance. High-tech care and specialists are concentrated in the large urban centers, as they are in many high-income countries. The private system tends to provide nicer amenities and shorter wait times than the public counterpart.

- **New Zealand**: Single-payer, government funded. Government at national and regional levels is heavily involved. General taxes fund most healthcare. A third of the residents have private insurance to pay uncovered services and copayments. There are private hospitals but public hospitals predominate, providing all emergency and intensive care.

- **Norway**: Single-payer, government-funded by general and payroll taxes. A tenth of the population pays for private insurance, mainly for quicker access and broader choice of providers. Most hospital care is provided at public, state-owned hospitals. There is a small private supplemental insurance market, mostly provided by employers.

- **Singapore**: Mixed financing. MediShield Life is a statutory insurance system that covers large hospital bills and certain costly outpatient treatments. (In the U.S., we'd call this catastrophic care.) Premiums for MediShield Life are subsidized by the government based on income and funded by general taxation. Patients pay premiums, deductibles, and co-insurance.

A second major program is called MediSave, a mandatory medical savings account that helps pay out-of-pocket expenses. MediSave accounts are tax-exempt and interest-bearing, funded by personal and employer contributions. Singapore utilizes regulation of supply and prices of health care services in the country to keep costs in check. There is a 50:50 mix of private and public hospital, the latter being government-owned. Sixty to 70% of citizens also have supplemental health insurance for coverage of private hospitals or private wards of public hospitals.

- **South Korea**: Single-payer, government-funded. Compulsory social insurance, called National Health Insurance, is funded largely by payroll taxes split equally between employers and employees. The national government also contributes. Co-payments for hospital care are 20% and outpatient services have co-payments ranging from 30 to 60%. Out-of-pocket payments are ~35% of national health expenditures, perhaps the highest of OECD countries. Out-of-pocket payments are capped, based on income. A large majority of the population also pays for private health insurance to help with co-payments. Low-income folks are in the Medical Aid Program and exempt from premiums and co-payments. Most hospitals are privately owned, but not-for-profit by law. Drug prices are set by the government.

- **Sweden**: Single-payer, government-funded.

Nearly all hospitals are public. Only 15% of healthcare expenditures are private, mostly out-of-pocket for dental care and drugs. There's a small market for supplemental insurance, mostly employer-provided, to gain quick access to specialists or to avoid wait lists for elective services.

· **Switzerland**: Mandatory private insurance bought from nonprofit insurers. Adults pay yearly deductibles and 10% coinsurance (with a cap) for all services. Care is largely decentralized, with system governance mainly at the cantonal level. Enrollees are offered several models of care (e.g., HMOs, Family Practice Gatekeeper, call-center before seeing physician) and a choice of deductibles. Funding is from enrollee premiums, taxes, other social insurance schemes (military, old-age, disability), and out-of-pocket. The Federal government and cantons subsidize premiums for lower-income individuals and households.

· **United Kingdom**: Single-payer socialized medicine. About 10% of residents have private supplementary insurance to gain more rapid access to elective care, choice of specialists, and better amenities.

· **United States**: Mixed public and private. Single-payer if 65 or older (Medicare, funded partly by payroll tax). Public insurance for no- or low-income under 65 (Medicaid). Private insurance. Out-of-pocket. Government sources pay for

~45% of total healthcare expenditures.

For additional details of 20 high-income country healthcare systems, check out The Commonwealth Fund's Country Profiles: International Health Care System Profiles (98). I note that many of these systems, perhaps a majority, provide free or very-low-cost medical education for physicians. They also limit the number of physicians trained, and limit the number of specialists. I also noticed that physicians in the U.S. tend to be paid significantly more than in many other top-tier countries. Other sources indicate that our nurses are paid more, too.

HOW DO CITIZENS OF OTHER COUTRIES RATE THEIR HEALTHCARE SYSTEMS?

It would be interesting to check healthcare system *satisfaction levels of residents* in high-income countries: Australia, Canada, France, Germany, Netherlands, New Zealand, Norway, Sweden, Switzerland, United Kingdom, and United States.

I'll stipulate at the outset that it is very difficult to find accurate, up-to-date, numbers on healthcare system satisfaction, particularly comparing one country to another. I found one survey (96) in which 25-30% of respondents were "neither satisfied nor dissatisfied." Furthermore, accuracy of satisfaction surveys can be affected by bias of the surveyors, source of the funds paying for the survey, specific wording of questions, number and economic class of survey participants, etc.

But first let's consider satisfaction in the U.S. based on data from a 2023 Gallup poll (95). Surveyed residents rated the overall *quality* of healthcare as excellent (10%), good (36%), or only fair (34%). They rated *coverage* as excellent (5%), good (25%), or only fair (37%). Regarding the healthcare industry as a business, 49% of respondents had a somewhat negative (31%) or very negative (18%) view. Regarding *cost* of the system, 19% were satisfied, 81% were dissatisfied. When asked if the system was in crisis or had major problems, 14% said "in crisis," 55% said "major problems," and these numbers were fairly steady over the prior 20 years. When asked if they preferred a government-run system versus one based on private insurance, 54% said private insurance, 44% preferred government-run. So even if you prefer socialized medicine, a majority of U.S. residents is not on board, at least not yet.

Ipsos in 2023 (97) published a multinational survey that touched on healthcare satisfaction. Unfortunately for us, the 28 countries did not include New Zealand, Norway, or Switzerland. Ipsos asked residents to "rate the *quality* of healthcare that you and your family have access to in your country." Options included "very good/good" and "very poor/poor." (You may well argue that the general public is in no position to judge the quality of their healthcare.) The global country average response of "very good/good" was 42%. Here are the "very good/good" responses by country:

- Australia: 64%
- United States: 61%
- Netherlands: 58%
- Sweden: 56%
- Great Britain: 48%

- Canada: 44%
- Germany: 41%
- France: 39%

Malaysia, by the way, was the top performer at 66%. Singapore was #4 at 63%. Most of the countries had a 25-30% "no opinion" gap between good and poor quality. You'll note several mentions of Malaysia in these survey results; I suspect respondents were in urban areas, and the rural residents would not be so positive. I'm sure you recall that in Chapter 1 of this snoozefest, the Legatum Prosperity Index's health pillar ranked Malaysia #42 out of 167 countries. You have been playing close attention, right? RIGHT?

Ipsos asked "How satisfied are you with the government's healthcare *policies*?" These are the "very/fairly satisfied" responses (the global country average was 48% "very/fairly satisfied"):

- Australia: 67%
- Netherlands: 62%
- Canada: 52%
- Germany: 50%
- United States: 45%
- Great Britain: 45%
- Sweden: 45%
- France: 36%

Singapore was tops at 81%.

Ipsos asked respondents to agree or not that it was *easy to get an appointment* with a local doctor. Here's the % that "strongly/tend to agree" (global country average was

39%);

- Netherlands: 55%
- United States: 48%
- Australia: 47%
- Sweden: 37%
- Canada: 35%
- Germany: 33%
- Great Britain: 29%
- France: 25%

India won at 62%.

Next, Ipsos asked if respondents agreed or not with, "I *trust* the healthcare system in my country to provide me with the best treatment." Global country average of "strongly/tend to agree" was 42%. Our residents at hand that "strongly/tend to agree:

- Australia: 58%
- Netherlands: 54%
- France: 48%
- Great Britain: 46%
- Sweden: 45%
- Canada: 44%
- Germany: 44%
- Unites States: 43%

Singapore and Malaysia were top of the chart at 63 and 61%, respectively.

More Ipsos poll questions:

Agree or disagree?: "*Waiting times* to get an appointment

with doctors *are too long* in my country." Global average for "strongly/tend to agree" was 60%. Here are "agrees" in our countries:

- Great Britain: 76%
- France: 68%
- Canada: 67%
- Germany: 65%
- Sweden: 61%
- Netherlands: 56%
- Australia: 55%
- United States: 42%

Agree or disagree?: "The healthcare system in my country is *overstretched*." Global average for "strongly/tend to agree" was 56%. Our countries:

- Great Britain: 83%
- Sweden: 79%
- France: 75%
- Netherlands: 71%
- Australia: 70%
- Canada: 69%
- Germany: 62%
- United States: 52%

Japan won this contest with only 14% thinking their system was overstretched.

Not surveyed by Ipsos were residents of New Zealand, Norway, and Switzerland.

In 2023 a satisfaction survey of Swiss adults found that

63% rated quality of care as very good or excellent (102). That percentage was 74 in 2020. Regarding medical care by their "regular doctor," 89% responded that it was very good or excellent. However, 60% noted it was somewhat or very difficult to get care on weekends, evenings, or holidays without going to an emergency department. (Isn't that an issue everywhere?) One out of every four adults had visited an ED in the prior two years. A quarter of the adults admitted foregoing a medical service (most often a doctor visit) due to the cost. Similar to France and Netherlands, Switzerland's chronic disease burden is somewhat lower than that in the U.S. and Australia.

Regarding system satisfaction in New Zealand, a Gallup World Poll in 2018 asked citizens "if they were satisfied with the availability of quality healthcare in the city or area where they lived." OECD reported that 82% of New Zealand citizens reported they were satisfied (103). The average citizen satisfaction response for all OECD countries was 70% in 2018. For comparison, the satisfaction number for Netherlands was 90%, Norway 89%, Switzerland 88%, Australia 86%, Germany 81%, Sweden 79%, U.S. 76%, Canada 75%, and France 69%. I was not able to find a more recent Gallup World Poll for all these countries other than 2018's.

A less extensive 2021 poll by OECD Trust Survey (104) asked citizens, "On a scale of 0 to 10, how satisfied or dissatisfied are you with the healthcare in [country] as a whole?" The "satisfied" responses for a few of our countries were South Korea 79%, Norway 77%, New Zealand 72%, France 64%, Sweden 57%, and Japan 51%. The average for OECD overall was 62%.

LESSONS LEARNED FROM CONSIDERING THE SYSTEMS OF OTHER COUNTRIES

After wading into the weeds of these mind-numbing satisfaction numbers, we find only a few clues about how we might devise a better system for the U.S. We can't necessarily conclude that a single-payer, social insurance, or private insurance systems is better than all others. **Many high-income countries have a mixture of public and private insurance, plus significant out-of-pocket costs, just like the U.S.** Whether single-payer, social insurance, or private insurance predominates, most countries have supplemental private- or employer-based insurance to help cover co-pays, dental care, drugs, out-of-pocket costs, and other non-covered services. Many non-U.S. systems use a variety of methods to control healthcare costs, such as:

- Limit the numbers of physicians and specialists, and the doctors earn less than U.S. doctors. Medical school tuition is free or minimal compared to the U.S. If you limit the supply of something like physicians, the price for services usually goes up. Supply and demand, etc. This may be why many countries set physician fee schedules, i.e., price controls. The risk of reducing income of U.S. physicians is that the smarter students will enter a different field with higher pay.

- Limit the numbers of hospitals and clinics, at least the public ones. Again, I'm not sure how this limits healthcare costs. I suppose if you use government money to build and run hospitals and clinics, you want them running near full capacity for the sake of efficiency. So limit the private facilities that could divert patients from the public system.

· Set healthcare fees. E.g., for physicians, hospitals, drugs.

· Negotiate the best drug prices from the suppliers and establish drug formularies based on cost-effectiveness and efficiency. E.g, if eight cholesterol-lowering statin drugs are on the market but all equally effective and safe, the formulary only carries one of the drugs, bought at a volume discount from the maker. They also utilize "external reference pricing" (117).

· Utilize co-pays and balance billing to help limit utilization and encourage healthful behaviors

· Allow physicians to have a private practice even if they also work in the public system. The private practice is an opportunity for supplemental income. Social insurance may still pay for private healthcare, but with higher co-pays and out-of-pocket costs.

· Utilize both public and private hospitals (the latter often not-for-profit by law). Social insurance may still pay for private healthcare, but with higher co-pays and out-of-pocket costs.

Most countries have a two-tier system, whereby you get more or "better" services if you can pay more, whether out-of-pocket or via private insurance. "Better" services could be shorter wait times, physically nicer facilities, less harried providers, a private hospital room, etc.

I had heard good things about the Singapore system before; Malaysia was a complete surprise (of course, it's right next door to Singapore). Australia and Netherlands are looking pretty good, too. U.K., Germany, and France may not be the best countries for the U.S. to emulate. We may also see some of the downsides to socialized medicine, such as difficulty getting a timely appointment with a physician. I often hear anecdotal horror stories about waiting months or years for a medical service you can get next week in the U.S. Nevertheless, the U.S. stands out as paying too much for healthcare.

As you think about healthcare reform, keep the Iron Triangle (99) in mind:

> The "Iron Triangle" of healthcare, often referred to in public health policy, consists of **cost**, **quality**, and **accessibility**. Alternatively, some scholars refer to equity (access by need and not by ability to pay), efficiency (generating incentives to reduce costs and improve quality), and cost as the "Iron Triangle" of healthcare. The most ideal public health policy is achieved when the three components are balanced. In other words, if a country's healthcare is sustainable, it can be assumed that the tensions in the three areas are being maintained at an optimal level. However, paradoxically, this means that improvements in one aspect of healthcare will always affect the other two. Therefore, for maintaining the sustainability of healthcare, it is crucial to balance the "Iron Triangle" by analyzing the current healthcare environment and supplementing the deficiencies.

We must also recognize that any healthcare system must dovetail to some degree with that country's history, culture, politics, and wealth level. Until the last 50 or 100 years, the U.S. had a strong history of self-reliance, freedom from government meddling, "live and let live" attitude, free-market capitalism, independence, inventiveness, respect for hard work, desire for justice, charity, Christianity, and sense of community. Vestiges of those remain. Those attitudes, along with abundant natural resources, once made our country great. Yet I can also understand the impulse to imagine healthcare as a sort of public utility, like water and sewer service, highways, the military, the electrical grid, and fire departments. After all, each one of us is going to get sick or injured someday and will need healthcare, ready and waiting. No matter how rugged an individual you are, you can't do high-tech healthcare on your own.

Healthcare reform will have to involve state and federal politicians. After all, they got us into this mess to begin with. Health insurers are regulated at both state and federal levels. State insurance commissioners will have to be involved. Don't worry about the burden on politicians and regulators; this is what we pay them to do. Your U.S. congressman has over 10 full-time staff, and senators have dozens, depending on their states' population. Annual salary of federal lawmakers is $174,000. Let them hash out the details of reform. I'll serve as a consultant.

Don't feel bad about asking your federal representatives to work. From OpenSecrets.org (45):

> More than half of those in Congress are millionaires, data from lawmakers' most recent personal financial disclosures shows. The median net worth of members of Congress who filed disclosures last year is just over $1 million.

Much of the wealth in Congress is concentrated at the top. The top 10 percent of wealthiest lawmakers have three times more wealth than the bottom 90 percent. While some lawmakers are still paying off student loans, others have paid off their third or fourth mortgage. The group of wealthiest members includes both career politicians who boosted their portfolios over decades in Congress and recently elected lawmakers.

* * *

The leaders of both chambers make the top 10 list [2020 data]. House Speaker Nancy Pelosi (D-Calif.) has seen her wealth increase to nearly $115 million from $41 million in 2004, the first year OpenSecrets began tracking personal finances. Senate Majority Leader Mitch McConnell (R-Ky.) saw his net worth increase from $3 million to over $34 million during that time. Both political leaders are married to affluent individuals who are driving those increases.

I am about to propose some ideas that may sound radical to you. But keep in mind that if all or most of my recommendations are followed, healthcare will be much less expensive than currently. I.e., the percentage of GDP devoted to healthcare will drop from 17.3% to 5%. Prices will drop by 70-75% on average. That means things that are out-of-reach unaffordable now can be paid for *outside of insurance*.

HERE'S WHAT WE NEED TO DO IN THE U.S.

1. Institute Price Transparency

Enact laws or regulations to this effect:

> All providers must post in their offices and on a public website a complete price list which will apply to every person, whether insured or self-pay. These prices are accepted as payment in full. All providers must have personnel available immediately to divulge prices of services and goods delivered or proposed. No one, including insurers, will ever have to pay more than the posted price.

The price list must be reasonably searchable and in terms a lay person can understand. If you are a provider and charge for band-aids, sutures, aspirin, or checking vital signs, you must list the price. Everything the provider charges for must be listed, along with the paid-in-full cash price. If it's not posted, there's no charge.

"Providers" are physicians, nurse practitioners, physician assistants, medical clinics, pharmacies, physical therapists, hospitals, emergency departments, urgent care centers, radiology facilities, laboratories and other diagnostic facilities, DME (durable medical equipment) providers, etc. A provider is every individual and every entity that provides a healthcare good or service and who holds themselves out as open to the public.

As an individual consumer you'll never pay more than the posted prices. You're free to negotiate a lower rate on your own.

As a provider, you can change your prices any time you like, but the price applies to everybody and you must post the prices online and at your site of delivery. You can charge more for weekends, holidays, night-times, emergency, and "rush orders." Just post the prices. You want to run a temporary "10% off on prostate exams" sale? Post the prices.

With price transparency, 270 million savvy consumers will be comparison shopping for best prices on initial office visits, chest x-rays, vaccinations, hernia repairs, lab work, colonoscopies, cardiac catheterizations, joint replacements, etc.

All customers must be given an itemized invoice listing actual charges for services and/or products at the time of delivery. The only exception is for services delivered over multiple consecutive days, such as hospitalizations, nursing homes, skilled nursing facilities, and rehabilitation centers. Those "multiple consecutive day" providers must provide a written initial good-faith estimate range (the ultimate bill for which CANNOT exceed the high-range estimate.

The customer is responsible for paying the charges. The customer can file a claim for reimbursement from the insurer, if one is involved, or the provider may volunteer to file the claim on the customer's behalf.

Noncompliant providers must be heavily penalized.

This means no more Medicare-specific or insurance-negotiated prices.

Mandated price transparency may require individual state and/or federal legislation. Or in the worst case scenario, a federal constitutional amendment. I say "worst case" because such amendments are very difficult to pass.

As of January or July, 2021, hospitals have been required

by federal regulation to list prices of at least 300 "shoppable services" on the Internet (70). Seventy of the services are mandates, and the hospital chooses the other 230 services. The American Hospital Association fought the regulation but lost the initial court case and the appeal. This is only a start.

2. Minimize Third-party Interference in the Patient-Provider Relationship

The interlopers include 1) insurance companies, 2) government (politicians and the regulators and bureaucrats empowered by them), 3) employers who enable insurance coverage, 4) employers of providers.

If you have a good and trusted healthcare provider, you need very little input from third parties.

We have to return to traditional indemnity health insurance, which operates just like your automobile insurance, homeowners insurance, and renter's insurance. This minimizes the third-party interference of insurance companies. Remember, none of their employees work for free, and the owners need a profit. You're paying for that; why pay more than necessary? Here's how indemnity works. You have a contract with a health insurance company that specifies they will compensate you for certain medical expenses you incur, in return for your premiums paid on a regular basis. This is indemnification. Let's say you're having chest pain so you see a provider and they charge you for a mid-level office visit, chest x-ray, and EKG (electrocardiogram or heart tracing). You pay the provider up front, then submit a claim for reimbursement with the insurance company. Or the provider may volunteer to file the claim for you. Whether you get reimbursed anything at all depends on your contract with the insurer. You may get zero reimbursement, or just 50%, 80%, or 100% of the billed amount. If your insurance company doesn't fulfill their end of the bargain, file a complaint with the state insurance commission. If that fails, you sue the insurer for breach of contract and lambaste them on social media, not necessarily in that order. This is how many other types of true insurance work.

Is your auto insurance, homeowners insurance, or renter's insurance linked to your current job? Do you lose those when you change jobs? Of course not. Health insurance should be the same. It only got linked to the workplace around the time of World War II because the federal government froze wages. Employers couldn't compete for talented workers on the basis of salary, but they could offer benefits such as health insurance. The rest is history. Another example of third-party interference.

If you have homeowners insurance and your house burns down, the insurer compensates you with some of the premium money that others have sent in for years, but never had a fire. This is exactly how insurance is designed to work. Not many houses burn down, but if it's your house, it's a catastrophe. All of us agree that healthcare is a vital part of our culture. After all, we all need it at some point. "Good health is true wealth." Health insurance makes expensive care available to those who aren't wealthy, by sharing the risk. When society agrees on a widespread social benefit, it's appropriate to subsidize that benefit via tax law. That's why employers get a tax deduction for health insurance premiums paid on behalf of their workers. But if a person is self-employed or their employer doesn't offer health insurance, she has to go to what is called the "individual market." Premiums are often much higher in the individual market, and purchasers get no tax break whatsoever. If her premium is $1,000/month, she has to earn ~$1,400/month because she has to pay $400/month in taxes to – you guessed it – the government. She's paying income tax AND payroll taxes (Medicare and Social Security).

We have ways to promote individually-owned insurance policies. Let's encourage (mandate?) them by making premiums free of income and payroll taxes, just like employer-provided insurance. One way to do that is by making the premiums deductible (as they are for employers), because healthcare is that important. Or institute a federal tax credit for folks in the individual insurance market. Insurance should follow us from job to job and through unemployment and retirement. See discussion of Health Savings Accounts (HSAs) under Miscellaneous Action Points below.

One popular effect of Obamacare is that it eliminated the problem of "pre-existing conditions." Prior to Obamacare, if you had a chronic condition such as diabetes, heart disease, or invasive cancer but lost your insurance coverage, it was then very expensive to replace your insurance coverage, if you could get any coverage at all. The insurer knew you were likely to be a high healthcare utilizer, costing them money. But pre-existing conditions were a problem primarily because healthcare is so damn expensive in this country. My recommended reforms to the healthcare system will greatly reduce costs. And if you developed diabetes, heart disease, or cancer while insured, the insurer should be on the hook to pay for related expenses for the rest of your life. Insurance companies base the premiums they charge on the odds you will or won't get sick. They win some bets, they lose others. State-based insurance commissioners must ensure that insurers in their state have the resources to pay those lost bets, and not simply file for bankruptcy.

Another popular feature of Obamacare is that it curtailed, if not eliminated, the insurance industry's tradition of medical underwriting. Medical underwriting refers to an insurer's setting premium rates based on an estimate of how much an individual was going to cost the insurer over the short- or long-term. For instance, a 60-year-old obese sedentary hypertensive smoker would have to pay a much higher premium than a healthy 20-year-old marathon-runner. You don't have to be a certified actuary to know which of these is likely to utilize the most healthcare services over the next 10 years. If you've ever bought a term life insurance policy, you've seen the same medical underwriting. In fact, all true insurance requires underwriting. If you have a poor driving record and live in a high auto-theft area, you're going to pay more for car insurance. That's underwriting. Until a Republican Congress gutted the Obamacare insurance-purchase mandate, the 20-year-old marathon-runner was subsidizing the 60-year-old's bad habits. Was that fair? Did that subsidy help motivate the 60-year-old to get healthy? No, it facilitated an unhealthy lifestyle. Again, if we reduce the overall cost of healthcare drastically, the insurers can return to their time-honored and logical medical underwriting.

Future federal legislators have the option of repealing or eliminating other parts of Obamacare. What do we do about pre-existing conditions then? Individually-owned policies may be the only fair way to approach it. Pre-existing conditions are a problem when the consumer changes jobs, loses their insurance because they quit paying premiums, employer changes the coverage, etc. When that happens, a patient loses their employer-provided insurance. The new employer-sponsored insurer may decline to cover a particular illness as a pre-existing condition. If an individual owns the policy, on the other hand, and a catastrophic event happens, the insurance company should be on the hook for life. If I get lung cancer, the insurer has lost their bet on me. They own that lung cancer for the rest of my life. Let's make individually-owned health insurance cancellable by the insurance company only for non-payment of premium or fraud by the policy holder. We could place caps on insurance premium increases, perhaps linked to the inflation rate.

Another source of onerous and costly third-party interference in healthcare is excessive regulation by federal bureaucrats. In 2024, the Supreme Court of the U.S. opened up an avenue for fighting this by overturing the "Chevron precedent." To explain this, I must remind you of something you learned in fifth grade civics class (at least back when they still taught civics). Our federal government has three branches: executive, legislative, and judicial. Each branch has responsibilities defined by the Constitution that are not to be encroached upon by the other branches. This is called "separation of powers." For instance, the legislative branch is responsible for writing and passing federal laws. The executive branch is responsible for enforcing (administrating) those laws, whether or not they agree with them. Now, note that federal legislators are not very bright, so they often write laws that are vague and ambiguous, then turn implementation of the law over to the executive (administrative) branch. The administrators then write regulations that interpret and implement what they thought the lawmakers were trying to do, too often going beyond the intent of Congress. Remember, the source of the problem in the first place is poorly written law. Administrative regulations have the force of law. If someone sues (in the judicial branch!) the executive branch for bureaucratic over-reach or mis-interpretation of the law, the "Chevron precedent" allows the court to tell the executive branch "just give us some reason, any reason, why you think your regulation is lawful and we'll probably go along with it." This is complicated, so here's an illustrative example from Contemplations on the Tree of Woe (118):

> Imagine Congress passes a new statute that gives the imaginary Bureau of Farm Regulation (BFR) the ability to regulate or ban "commercial products relating to dairy animals." The imaginary regulators at the BFR then publish their list of regulations, and among these regulations, the BFR bans the use of vegan leather (AKA pleather).
>
> The banning of pleather sends a shockwave through the fashion industry. A coalition of fashion labels led by Balenciaga sue the BFR, because their upcoming line of apparel is entirely made from vegan leather sourced from conflict-free sustainable petroleum

manufactories.

When the case goes to court, the BFR says "Pleather is a commercial substitute for leather in fashion, so therefore it relates to leather; leather is a commercial product made from cows, so therefore it relates to cows; and cows are dairy animals; therefore pleather is a commercial product relating to dairy animals, and we can ban it." Under the Chevron Doctrine, the Court hearing the case is forced to say "well BFR, since you have your reasons, you're good to go!"

Now ask yourself: By this reasoning, is there anything the BFR *couldn't ban*? "Cars are used to transport dairy products, therefore we can regulate cars." "Guns are used to shoot varmints that prey on animals that produce dairy products, therefore we can regulate guns." And so on.

With this (admittedly extreme) example, you can understand why the Chevron Doctrine was so important to the power of the Deep State. It effectively **insulated** all the regulatory agencies from judicial review and enabled them to act with virtually unchecked power. All they had to do was offer some reason for their regulation.

This Chevron Doctrine (aka Chevron deference) allowed the executive (administrative) branch to essentially make laws by giving their own interpretation of legislative intent. The Supreme Court in 2024 sort of said this violates the Constitutional separation of powers. The legislative branch makes laws, not the executive branch. The Court actually wrote "The Administrative Procedure Act [of 1946] requires courts to exercise their independent judgment in deciding whether an agency has acted within its statutory authority, and courts may not defer to an agency interpretation of the law simply because a statute is ambiguous; Chevron is overruled." So when an administrating executive agency is sued for bureaucratic over-reach or law-making, the judicial branch has to make its own determination of the law rather than deferring to the agency's interpretation. Now, I don't have the resources to sue the executive branch. But I know who might: state and national medical societies, American Hospital Association, Big Pharma, medical device manufacturers, etc.

MEDICARE: WHAT TO DO ABOUT IT

Medicare is a federal insurance program for folks over 65, certain younger people with disabilities, and for those with end-stage renal disease. The different parts of Medicare help cover specific services:

- **Medicare Part A (Hospital Insurance)**
  Part A covers inpatient hospital stays, care in a skilled nursing facility, hospice care, and some home health care.

- **Medicare Part B (Medical Insurance)**
  Part B covers certain doctors' services (including most doctor services if you're in a hospital), outpatient care, medical supplies, preventive services, ambulance services, and both outpatient and inpatient mental health.

- **Medicare Part D (prescription drug coverage)**
  Helps cover the cost of prescription drugs

(including many recommended shots or vaccines).

Part A: Most Medicare enrollees don't pay a periodic premium for Part A. They or their spouses have been paying for it for decades as part of payroll taxes. For those who have to purchase Part A the monthly premiums in 2024 are $278 or $505, depending on how long they or their spouses paid into the program via payroll tax.

Part B: Every Medicare enrollee pays a monthly premium for Part B. In 2024, that standard amount is $174.70. Those with recent income above a certain level pay more. If you're on Social Security, the monthly premium is automatically deducted from your benefit check. In 2024, the Medicare Part B deductible is $240. After that, you only pay for 20% of the Medicare-approved amount for covered services. Yes, this is government fee-setting.

Part D: Medicare drug coverage helps pay for prescription drugs you need. To get Medicare drug coverage, you must join a Medicare-approved plan that offers drug coverage (this includes Medicare drug plans and Medicare Advantage Plans with drug coverage). Each plan can vary in cost and specific drugs covered, but must give at least a standard level of coverage set by Medicare. Medicare drug coverage includes generic and brand-name drugs. Plans can vary the list of prescription drugs they cover (called a formulary) and how they place drugs into different "tiers" on their formularies. Plans have different monthly premiums. You'll also have other costs throughout the year in a Medicare drug plan. How much you pay for each drug depends on which plan you choose.

Certain Medicare plans, such as Medicare Advantage, have different rules but must give you at least the same coverage as original Medicare. From Medicare's website:

Medicare Advantage is an "all in one" alternative to Original Medicare. These "bundled" plans include Part A, Part B, and usually Part D. Most plans offer extra benefits that Original Medicare doesn't cover — like vision, hearing, dental, and more. Medicare Advantage Plans have yearly contracts with Medicare and must follow Medicare's coverage rules. The plan must notify you about any changes before the start of the next enrollment year.

Whether Medicare is constitutional is debatable. It establishes the federal government as the largest single insurer in the country. I can't imagine our country's founders agreeing that this was a proper role of the government rather than private businesses. Created in 1965, the Medicare program was likely deemed constitutional on the basis of the general welfare or commerce clauses. Or the constitution was simply ignored, as it so often has been. The same clauses today could be used to justify socialized housing and food. Lack of housing and food will kill you quicker than lack of health insurance. Nevertheless, the Medicare program is with us for the foreseeable future. I favor phasing Medicare out (and the Medicare payroll tax) eventually, replacing it with true indemnity insurance, charity, health savings accounts, and Medicaid for the needy.

One way to improve the Medicare program in the near-term would be to eliminate the government price controls that pay the best and worst providers the same amount. Medicare should institute "reference pricing," specifying in advance how much they will pay for a given service, regardless of what the provider charges. The patient can either pay the difference (called balance billing), decline the service and find a different provider, or obtain additional private insurance coverage. This would immediately facilitate competition by providers for Medicare patients. As we have seen in so many sectors of the economy, competition improves service and lowers cost.

The administrative burden of Medicare on the providers can be alleviated by repealing claims-filing requirements. Medicare has a form for patients to file their own claims. Medicare can then reimburse the Medicare patient directly for all claims.

The following is an esoteric point that will only apply to a few people. Let's say you're getting Social Security benefits. Let's stipulate further that although you become eligible for Part A when you reach age 65, but you want to turn down Part A coverage, perhaps because you're one of the few people who have to pay monthly premiums for Part A, and you have access to less expensive or better coverage elsewhere. If you turn down Part A, your Social Security benefit will be cut off (62). That would hurt most people financially. If our rulers would allow citizens to dis-enroll from Part A without foregoing Social Security payments, it would immediately decrease government spending and facilitate a true insurance market for those over 65.

MEDICAID AND CHIP: WHAT TO DO ABOUT THEM

We are a rich, charitable country. We will not tolerate patients dying in the streets after months of suffering for lack of healthcare or the funds to pay for it. We will provide a safety net for the needy. Medicaid and CHIP (Children's Health Insurance Program) are major threads in that net. These programs for low-income folks are jointly funded by state and federal governments.

Allow me to introduce you to the principle of subsidiarity (63):

> This tenet holds that nothing should be done by a larger and more complex organization which can be done as well by a smaller and simpler organization. In other words, any activity which can be performed by a more decentralized entity should be. This principle is a bulwark of limited government and personal freedom. It conflicts with the passion for centralization and bureaucracy characteristic of the Welfare State.

Have you noticed that the federal government has relatively little say in how our public schools are run? If the U.S. Department of Education were abolished overnight, the only thing you'd notice is reduction in your federal taxes. All the major players in public schools are local: students, parents, teachers, support staff, nearly all funding, school board members, superintendents, even businessmen who will need graduates to work for them. It would be pure folly for Anadarko (Oklahoma) Public Schools to be run by Washington, D.C., politicians. They don't know jack about Anadarko. Anadarko Public Schools runs the show, in accordance with the principle of subsidiarity.

In terms of medical care, the subsidiarity principle means that politicians and bureaucrats in the District of Columbia shouldn't be in charge of indigent (or any other) healthcare in North Dakota, Louisiana, and Vermont. Those states' citizens are in a much better position to care for their poor. The locals know their particular causes of poverty, know the best ways to counteract poverty, know what's culturally acceptable, can keep a closer eye on the programs, can make quicker adjustments, etc.

Federal Medicaid funds should be block-granted to the states, eventually phasing out federal dollars entirely (with a concomitant reduction in federal tax rates!). States will use their own money for healthcare of their indigent citizens. States that do a great job will be examples for the laggards. Local control is nearly always better than distant.

OTHER INTERFERING THIRD PARTIES

In 2022, 74% of U.S. physicians were employed by hospitals, health systems, or other corporate entities (64). That compares to 47% in 2018. An employer can be an interfering 3rd party. For one example, see my prior discussion on the overutilization of subspecialty care versus primary care (#17 in causes of expensive care).

Finally, let's not forget another third party in the exam room with you and your doctor: lawyers. Predatory personal injury lawyers are always in the back of your physician's mind, ready to pounce at the hint of an unfavorable outcome. The practice of "defensive medicine" by physicians accounts for at least two or three percent of total healthcare costs. The defense is against malpractice lawsuits.

Are there ways to reduce the financial toll of malpractice lawsuits on providers? One method that has worked in some states is a regulatory financial cap on damages ($) payable to plaintiffs (injured patients or their survivors). For example, California has capped non-economic damages ("pain and suffering") at $250,000. If set at an appropriate level, such caps also make some cases less attractive to trial lawyers.

Another possible solution would be to institute the "English Rule," by which the legal costs of both parties are allocated to the losing party. Texas (in 2011) and Alaska have some form of this rule. To be workable, the English Rule would probably also require some assurance that the loser will be able to pay those legal costs. Such assurance could take the form of insurance or existing pledged assets. The English Rule would tend to discourage plaintiffs who have weak cases and are motivated solely by greed or vindictiveness.

Yet another idea is "health courts" specializing in medical malpractice. I assume these would leave lay juries out of these complicated cases, similar to how workers' compensation cases don't involve juries.

MISCELLANEOUS ACTION POINTS

Repeal certificate-of-need laws.

Return all regulation of the provision of healthcare and health insurance to the states, consistent with the principle of subsidiarity (63) and the U.S. Constitution (what used to be called "the supreme law of the land"). States already have regulatory bodies overseeing physicians, pharmacists, nurses, physical therapist, hospitals, insurance companies, etc.

Allow physician-owned hospitals again.

Repeal claims-filing requirements for providers. Insurer reimburses the enrollee (patient) for paid claims.

Improve and encourage HSAs (health savings accounts). HSAs are savings accounts with your name on it because it's your money. The account follows you from job to job and into retirement. To qualify for an HSA you have to be signed up for a high-deductible insurance plan, be under age 65, and be able to save some money. Many employers will contribute to your account via payroll deduction with pre-tax dollars. So you save money on your taxes early on. Account deposits don't necessarily have to come from your employer. If you fund the account with after-tax dollars, those dollars are a deduction on your current years' income, so more savings on taxes. The maximum savings contribution for an individual is $3,850 for an individual and $7,750 for a family in 2023. If over 55 years of age, an additional $1,000 is allowed. The savings are used to pay out-of-pocket expenses like deductibles and co-pays for a variety of medical, mental health, and dental services; even feminine hygiene products. Most HSAs give you a debit card to pay your medical expenses. Money left over at the end of the year rolls over into the next year. Withdrawals for qualified medical expenses are free from federal and most state taxes. These accounts can even be used as investment vehicles with tax-free earnings. If you withdraw money for non-qualified purposes before age 65, you'll owe income tax and a 20% penalty. Money withdrawn for non-medical expenses after age 65 are subject only to income tax. Current HSAs are perhaps best for those who don't anticipate major medical expenses in the near future. With legislative modification, HSAs could be widely used as a substitute for employer-provided health insurance. Initial modifications might be to increase the contribution limits and allow HSA money to pay health insurance premiums.

Repeal any regulations that prevent insurers and employers from designing affordable plans (e.g., allow limited and catastrophic coverage).

Repeal overly restrictive state and federal mandates.

Repeal EHR (electronic health records) requirements. Let's trust the provider to choose the best record-keeping method.

Make premiums on private/individual policies deductible for income tax purposes.

Subsidize charity care via tax incentives.

Repeal EMTALA (Emergency Medical Treatment and Labor Act). This law forces emergency departments of hospitals that participate in Medicare to accept all patients, regardless of ability to pay. This means that hospitals and involved physicians are forced to provide "charity" care. Charity is voluntary by definition. Physicians don't even get a tax deduction for the value of this uncompensated care. We don't force grocers to give away free food to those in need. Instead, we have the food stamp program - SNAP or Supplemental Nutrition Assistance Program – to provide food for the indigent. The cost is borne by the general population via taxation. We don't force residential real estate owners to freely open their doors to the homeless and indigent. Instead, we have public housing and Section 8 rent assistance. The cost is borne by the general population via taxation. On the other hand, the financial burden of EMTALA falls directly on hospitals and physicians. Of course, those costs in part must be passed on to the more well-off patients. Otherwise the provider goes out of business. I propose tax deductions for providers who respond to true medical emergencies, when usual fee collection methods fail.

If Congress fails to repeal EMTALA, the fallback position is for the U.S. Treasury to pay providers their usual fees directly and promptly for uncompensated emergency care mandated by EMTALA.

Eliminate government price controls on physician fees (e.g., the Medicare Physician Fee Schedule). Public insurance programs (e.g., Medicare, Medicaid, Tricare) can no longer set the fees for providers. They can tell consumers how much the program will pay for something, such as a colonoscopy, but the provider determines what price to charge the consumer. Consumer then agrees, or shops elsewhere.

WHAT ABOUT CARE FOR THE INDIGENT?

The U.S.A. will never be without a safety net for those unable to pay for healthcare. We are a prosperous and charitable country. Americans gave $499 billion to charities in 2022 (65). A majority of donations went to religion (27%), human services (14%), education (13%), grant-making foundations (11%), and health (10%).

Herein, I'm including among the indigent those with no income and low income, plus those who have no- or low-income *and* no other assets of any sort to pay for care or insurance. If you have significant assets but no income, you need to sell your assets to pay for *your* care.

The first thing we need to do is drastically reduce the

cost of care as in this reform manifesto. Then you have more folks who can afford care whereas previously they were priced out of the market. Furthermore, citizens will have more money in their bank accounts for charitable donations.

Indigent care funding will come from a patchwork of sources, including:

- Family
- Churches, synagogues, mosques, and other religious organizations
- Charities
- Social crowd-funding
- Taxpayers

Let's look at taxpayer-funded Medicaid, a public health insurance program for low-income people which already covers one in four residents as of 2022. Also be aware of CHIP (Children's Health Insurance Program), a closely related program which is for children in low-come families and their parents. CHIP is co-funded by the feds and each state. Medicaid spending is 18% of national health expenditure; in other words, $1 of every $6 spent on healthcare in the U.S. Medicaid is funded jointly by the federal government and each state, with the feds contributing ~65% of the total. For most states, Medicaid is typically the single largest expenditure. K-12 education is the second largest.

So we're already spending a lot on indigent healthcare.

Who knows best how to care for the indigent population in your state? Politicians and paper-pushers in Washington, D.C, or the state and local leaders who live in your state year-round? Why on earth are Californians sending tax dollars to D.C. for distribution to Medicaid programs in Mississippi and West Virginia? Why not let Californians take care of their own indigent with their own tax dollars?

Here's my specific reform proposal for Medicaid. Reduce federal tax rates so that each states' taxpayers retain more money in their own state. Let the states use that "extra" money to run their Medicaid programs as they see fit, without federal intervention whatsoever. Yes, this means ending the federal portion of Medicaid. State and local leaders will likely do a better job at management. They are intimately familiar with local conditions and are more responsive to the citizens. States that do a poor job can learn from the well-run states. This reform is in line with the principles of federalism (see U.S. Constitution) and subsidiarity.

In this schema, individual states will decide if they want to fund healthcare for indigent illegal aliens. Detecting, monitoring, and deporting illegal aliens is the job of the federal government. If a states' citizens decline to provide healthcare for illegals, the federal government must reimburse the state for their healthcare and costs of deportation.

What about communities that have hospitals, clinics, or physicians that refuse to see indigent patients. I fully expect charities will step up to the plate and fill the need. This could include paying the healthcare bills or owning and staffing healthcare facilities.

3. Promote Competition Among Providers

To locate high-quality providers, consult your trusted

friends and relatives, physicians, nurses, pharmacists, even trial lawyers.

Check out your prospective provider at the appropriate state licensing authority.

Ask your Congressional representatives to open up the National Practitioner Data Bank to the public. From the NPDB website:

> The National Practitioner Data Bank (NPDB) is a web-based repository of reports containing information on medical malpractice payments and certain adverse actions related to health care practitioners, providers, and suppliers. Established by Congress in 1986, it is a workforce tool that prevents practitioners from moving state to state without disclosure or discovery of previous damaging performance.
>
> Federal regulations authorize eligible entities to report to and/or query the NPDB. Individuals and organizations who are subjects of these reports have access to their own information. The reports are confidential, and not available to the public.
>
> The NPDB assists in promoting quality health care and deterring fraud and abuse within health care delivery systems.

Check online reviews of providers.

Query local court records for lawsuits involving specific providers. Compare various providers but keep in mind the number of years in practice: the more years, the more exposure to lawsuits. And getting sued does not necessarily mean malpractice was committed. As of

2022, one in three physicians have been sued during their careers to date. Men are more likely than women to get sued. Certain specialties, like surgeons and ob-gyns are at significantly higher-than-average risk.

High-deductible ($2000-$5000) insurance policies for all. This puts skin in the game so consumers start shopping for the best deals. The deductible amount must be allowed to rise or fall, depending on inflation/deflation. Make it a percentage of median local household income?

4. Slash Administrative Costs

Billing and insurance-related costs are a major factor in overall healthcare costs.

There's a simple solution: The consumer pays the provider, then files a claim for reimbursement from his insurer. The provider may or may not volunteer to file the claim. If the insurer fails to pay a legitimate claim, the patient files a complaint with the state insurance commissioner and/or sues the insurer for breach of contract. Many of these issues could be handled in small claims court. Insurance companies love to deny payment of claims by providers because it increases their profits. They will soon tire of battling an angry consumer who has plenty of time to focus on one claim. If the insurer

defrauds too many consumers, the insurance commissioner will bring the hammer down. Private attorneys will also be interested in helping out.

Allow providers to simply state the condition that was evaluated or treated, rather than using ICD-10-CM codes. There are over 14,000 diagnosis codes in the

International Classification of Diseases, 10th Revision, Clinical Modification. Most, if not all, insurers require the use of these codes when a claim is submitted. Centers for Medicare and Medicaid publishes a 121-page guideline on how to use the codes (66). Just scan that link for a taste of the complexity. Providers and insurers employ clerks to ensure adherence. "Superficial scalp laceration, 2-inches long, repaired with five staples" should be adequate documentation. I wouldn't be surprised if ICD-19 has a specific code for that plus incorporating the mechanism of injury, infection present or not, foreign body present or not, which part of the scalp, and whether pediatric or adult.

It's reasonable for in insurer to require a diagnosis code. That's how they know if they're obligated to cover it. They also require a procedure code, also reasonable. With "superficial scalp laceration, 2-inches long, repaired with five staples," I've combined diagnosis and procedure codes. But our healthcare system isn't satisfied with that, and so requires a Current Procedural Terminology (CPT) code (67). A procedure can be an office visit, diagnostic test, surgery, etc. CPT is a classification system invented and copyrighted by the American Medical Association in 1966. I don't know how many procedure codes exist, but it's probably in the thousands. And they are revised yearly.

Healthcare providers and insurers employ legions of full-time workers to oversee billing and insurance-reimbursement. We need to simplify healthcare billing. The coders and clerks working in that sector will find more useful jobs in the broader economy.

5. Limit Lobbying By Well-Financed Organizations

The healthcare industry spends hundreds of millions of dollars on federal-level lobbying, and a smaller but not insignificant amount in the states. I don't know what those dollars actually pay for. I consider lobbying to be a form of free speech which is guaranteed by the Bill of Rights in the Constitution (1st amendment). So limiting lobbying is a conundrum. I need your ideas on this one. Electing honest, ethical, Constitution-honoring lawmakers would certainly help, and fire those who aren't. Severely punish politicians and bureaucrats who take bribes.

Approaches discussed in other sections will greatly reduce the obscene profits in the system, which will naturally reduce the money spent on lobbying.

Reducing government's third-party interference role in healthcare will also naturally reduce lobbying.

Lee Drutman at Governance Studies at Brookings has a proposal to make lobbying more transparent (48):

> The Library of Congress should create a website that will become the de facto online forum and clearinghouse for all public policy advocacy. Such a website would both level the playing field (it is much cheaper to post a web page than to hire an army of lobbyists to descend on Washington) and increase transparency and accountability (if all positions and arguments are public, everyone knows who is lobbying for what and why). This will result in more democratic

and more thoroughly vetted public policy.

With billions of dollars on the line, I suspect the players, including politicians, would quickly figure out a way to circumvent Drutman's system.

6. Deconstruct Monopolies

All antitrust, anti-competitive, and consumer protection laws must be vigorously enforced at both state and federal levels. Elect politicians who will enforce the laws already on the books. If district attorneys and attorneys general won't do it, private lawsuits with stiff penalties must be allowed.

Requiring a physician order to "allow" a patient to get a diagnostic test done is akin to a monopoly. It also tends to be anti-competitive. I propose that any test or diagnostic procedure that carries no exposure to drugs nor is invasive beyond a blood draw, may be purchased without a doctor's order or prescription. Same for diagnostic procedures that involve radiation or potentially harmful contrast media, as long as a radiologist at the facility approves the test after reviewing risks with the purchaser. Insurers can set restrictions on what they'll pay for, however. Consumers in Arizona already, for example, can order a great variety of blood tests, paying out of pocket. Thank you, Elizabeth Holmes (68).

Medicare and Medicaid are monopolies. They need to be transitioned to become regular health insurers so that their enrollees – the elderly, indigents, and the totally disabled - can choose from various other commercial insurers. Let the competition begin! Most folks on Medicare have already paid into the system over decades if they've had a job. The current Medicare tax on employee wages is 2.9%. If the government considers you highly-paid, the tax is even higher. As Medicare is phased out, so will be the tax. Some argue that Medicare is unconstitutional anyway.

Many hospitals and healthcare systems (including accountable care organizations) are monopolies. Particularly after the heavy consolidation (mergers, etc.) in the industry in the last couple decades. Break up these monopolies. Prevent new mergers and consolidations that are anti-competitive. The pharmaceutical field is also heading into anti-competitive consolidation, with insurers and pharmacies owning pharmacy benefits managers (PBMs).

Meredith P. Rosenthal, PhD, is with the Department of Health Policy and Management, Harvard T.H. Chan School of Public Health in Boston, MA. Rosenthal in a 2021 viewpoint article cites inadequate competition as the major driver of high out-of-pocket healthcare costs (74):

What steps can be taken to address rising out-of-pocket costs for people in the US with employer-sponsored insurance? First and most important, policy makers must address the fundamental drivers of health care price increases, foremost of which is the growth of market power among physician groups, hospitals, and health systems and consequent lack of adequate competition. In addition to increasing antitrust scrutiny of consolidation of practices and health care organizations and anticompetitive conduct, state and federal regulators could introduce limits on the levels or growth rates of the prices commercial insurers pay for health care. The political obstacles to passage of price controls are substantial, however, and federal price regulation seems out of reach at least in the immediate future. At a minimum, policy makers should continue to increase the availability of information about health care prices, including pharmaceutical rebates and administrative fees that are paid to pharmacy benefit managers, which have been implicated in recent out-of-pocket cost increases for insulin. While transparency alone has limited effectiveness as a cost-control tool, such information could increase the demand for more selective clinician or health care networks or steering tools such as reference pricing, while building the case for price regulation over the long term.

Eliminate certificate-of-need laws and regulations.

Allow wholesalers and individual citizens to purchase drugs from outside the U.S.

Fast-track the approval of generic drugs.

Allow Medicare and Medicaid, as long as they exist, to negotiate better drug prices for enrollees.

Enable and encourage the Federal Trade Commission to prosecute anti-competitive practices of non-profit organizations.

Do not allow public insurers to pay more for services in a hospital-owned "outpatient facility" as compared to a typical outpatient clinic not owned by a hospital.

In a way, requiring a physician's prescription in order to purchase a drug is a bit of medical monopoly. This makes the physician a potential third-party interloper, too. I'm sure that pharmacists and physicians could expand the list of drugs adequately safe for public access without a prescription.

7. Reduce Drug Prices

Price transparency will help greatly. Consumers who leave the doctor's office with a prescription will be able to go online and conveniently shop for the lowest price. Pharmacies will compete for the business.

End the safe harbor from anti-kickback law enjoyed by PBMs (Pharmacy Benefit Managers) and Group Purchasing Organizations. See 42 U.S.C. 1320a-7b(b)(c)(C) and 42 CFR 1001.952(j). This would decrease drug prices and cut the flow of money to middlemen who add no value to patient care.

Several think tanks have proposed that wholesale drug pricing in the U.S. must be on "most favored nation" basis. Meaning, if Merck sells a drug to the National Health Service in the UK at the lowest price of any country, they have to sell for same price in the U.S. I'm not sold on this idea yet. Do we really want the federal government setting prices, like it currently does for Medicare? Sounds unconstitutional.

Allow U.S. citizens and companies to import drugs from outside the U.S. and sell them here. There was a time long ago that we made the bulk of our medicines in the U.S. But now, 70% of the manufacturing facilities for our drugs are located elsewhere, particularly the European Union, India, and China (50). Yes, we need certain safeguards, etc. That's why we fund a Food and Drug Administration.

Streamline the process for converting drugs newly off-patent into the generic market.

If a drug or medical device is developed with use of *any* public money (taxpayer dollars), the usual patent and exclusivity lengths should not fully apply.

As long as Medicare and Medicaid are paying for drugs, allow them to negotiate prices with manufacturers and wholesalers.

SUMMARY OF MY RECOMMENDATIONS

My prescription for reform is a return to high-deductible major-medical indemnity insurance. Comparable to the insurance many of us already have on our automobiles and homes. You are the policyholder, not your employer, so insurance follows you from job to job to retirement. Price transparency will create 270,000,000 shoppers balancing cost and quality according to their individual needs. Additional cost savings and quality improvements will come from vibrant competition and massive curtailment of third-party meddling in the patient-provider relationship. Government regulation of healthcare and health insurance will be returned to the individual states, with minimization of mandates and maximization of freedom. In this optimal environment, technology, innovation, and competition will drastically reduce the cost of healthcare while improving quality.

If You Want to Help Make a Change RIGHT NOW

Here are some ideas:

- Contact your lawmakers with specific recommendations (demands?) and give them a copy of this book. Important examples follow...
- Insist on price transparency.
- Advocate a return to traditional indemnity health insurance that is not employer-based. With premiums exempt from payroll and income taxes. Insurance non-cancellable except for non-payment of premiums or fraud by the policyholder.
- Allow insurance companies to do medical underwriting.
- Until Medicare is phased-out, institute reference pricing and allow balance billing.
- Turn Medicaid funding and administration entirely over to the states.
- Return all regulation of the provision of healthcare and health insurance to the states.
- Improve and encourage HSAs (Health Savings Accounts).
- Minimize insurance mandates.
- Subsidize charity care via tax incentives to providers.
- Reduce administrative costs by paying your healthcare provider yourself then you file a claim for reimbursement from your insurer. Many providers will gladly file the initial simple claim for you.
- Either repeal EMTALA or give providers a tax credit for the charity care they provide.
- Insist that politicians, attorneys general, and the Federal Trade Commission enforce current antitrust and consumer protection laws, and

repeal anti-competitive laws.

- As long as Medicare and Medicaid are paying for drugs, allow them to negotiate prices with manufacturers and wholesalers.

And don't forget: Get yourself as healthy as possible so you can avoid the American medical-industrial complex. Lose that excess weight. Exercise regularly. Eat healthful food. Get science-based screening tests on schedule.

FALLBACK POSITIONS

Let's face it. I'm asking for a lot in this manifesto! It took decades for us to end up with our current system. It will take years to fix it, or even head it in the right direction. If the bulk of my recommendations prove unpopular or impossible to implement (which is likely), seriously consider these options:

- Mimic the Singapore system (111). It's highly ranked, allows for flexibility, and has many features Americans are already familiar with. Health Savings Accounts figure prominently. Singaporeans are happy with it. In 2016, Singapore's system ran on just 4.5% of GDP (gross national product). Really worth checking out. But we may not be smart enough to make that system work here: average IQ in Singapore is ~107 compared to 98 in the U.S.
- "Medicare for All." I didn't make that up; it's been under consideration for years (113, 114,115). In 2022, our three largest social insurance operations–Medicare, Medicaid, and CHIP–already accounted for almost 42% of

our national health expenditures (NHE) (112). (Medicare is 22.2% of NHE; Medicaid/CHIP is 19.5%.). These programs provide for nearly 40% of the population, 39.7% to be precise. Why not extend that coverage to the other 60% of us? It's a crazy idea, crazy enough that it just might work! Especially if we incorporated enough of my other recommendations.

EPILOGUE

Congratulations, dear reader, for slogging your way through this screed! I know it wasn't easy, exciting, entertaining, or sexy. But hopefully educational and motivational.

This was the most difficult writing project I've ever tackled. Starting about 60 years ago, our U.S. healthcare system has become an increasingly opaque, convoluted, and chaotic mess. I can't help thinking that "the powers that be" want it that way. It makes it easier for them to manipulate the system out of sight of the general public. The citizens who need great, affordable healthcare should be the major stakeholders in this enterprise. Instead, we are confused and manipulated pawns.

I mentioned earlier that reform will have to involve state and federal lawmakers. As the late, great H. L. Mencken put it:

> A professional politician is a professionally dishonorable man. In order to get anywhere near high office he has to make so many compromises and submit to so many humiliations that he becomes indistinguishable from a streetwalker.

At least a streetwalker delivers on her promises.

My favorite modern political commentator is P.J. O'Rourke, who died in 2022:

- "Giving money and power to government is like giving whiskey and car keys to teenage boys."
- "A little government and a little luck are necessary in life, but only a fool trusts either of them."
- "When buying and selling are controlled by legislation, the first things to be bought and sold are legislators."
- "It is a popular delusion that the government wastes vast amounts of money through inefficiency and sloth. Enormous effort and elaborate planning are required to waste this much money."
- "Politicians are wonderful people as long as they stay away from things they don't understand, such as working for a living."
- "A politician who portrays himself as 'caring' and 'sensitive' because he wants to expand the government's charitable programs is merely saying that he's willing to try to do good with other people's money."

But what do most Americans think about their

politicians? A 2022 poll by Pew Research Center (110) found that:

- Only 20% trust the federal government to do the right thing "just about always or most of the time."
- Only 8% describe the federal government as being responsive to the needs of ordinary Americans.
- Only 27% would say the federal government is doing well at being "careful with taxpayer money."
- Only 52% say they have confidence in career federal government workers (not political appointees) to act in the best interest of the public.
- Nevertheless, 69% support the federal government having a major role in ensuring access to healthcare.

The Pew report mentions that state and local governments are viewed more favorably (subsidiarity!):

About two-thirds (66%) say they have a favorable view of their local government, compared with 54% who have a favorable view of their state government and just 32% who have a favorable view of the federal government.

Am I optimistic that the healthcare system can be changed for the better? Remember, change will have to involve politicians, entrenched bureaucrats, and judges. Unfortunately, an overwhelming majority of our politicians (and many judges) are corrupt. The ones not corrupted by money or power are often controlled by blackmail. Where does the money come from? Lobbyists and bribery. Like the general population, some politicians are psychopaths, others are just plain evil. Generally, the higher the level of government, the more corrupt. Even when we vote apparently honest and moral lawmakers into office, once they get power, most of them change like chameleons. (If you're over 60, you need to recognize that the U.S. today is not the same country you grew up in although you may still regard with allegiance. That country is long gone.) If you don't think the U.S. is corrupt to some degree, note that Transparency International ranked the U.S. higher in corruption than Australia, Canada, U.K., France, Germany, Netherlands, New Zealand, Norway, Sweden, Switzerland, and Singapore (116). Setting aside city and state level corruption and incompetence, let's look at some of the things our federal politicians have done recently (and judges allowed):

- They created a taxation system that allows multi-millionaires and billionaires to pay much lower taxes, percentagewise, than the average middle- or upper middle-class wage-slave.
- They run a system whereby 75% of the country's wealth is owned by the top 10% of households.
- Out-of-control federal deficit spending has caused inflation that is hurting many of us and hobbling the economy, which will worsen if current trends continue. We will also see cutbacks in legitimate social spending.
- They bomb innocent civilians in multiple countries without declarations of war or the consent of the governed (us). They don't even consult us. If not doing the bombing, we provide the bombs or pay for the bombs.

- They meddle in foreign governments and elections where we have no legitimate right or business.
- They re-defined "marriage," so it's no longer a union between a man and a woman. The most recently appointed Supreme Court justice couldn't even define "woman" in her confirmation hearing (119).
- They opened the country's border so that literally anyone can come in and stay indefinitely, often at great expense to the taxpayers.
- They send billions of our taxpayer dollars to foreign countries without our consent or consultation.
- They imprison political dissidents who exercise their constitutional right to peaceably assemble and petition the government for a redress of grievances.
- They told us that Russia's 2022 attack on Ukraine was entirely unprovoked, but we learned much later of longstanding secret Central Intelligence Agency intelligence operations in Ukraine "in which the agency sponsored and built up the Ukrainian intelligence agency (HUR), using it as a weapon of spying, assassinations and other provocations directed against Russia for more than a decade." Per the *New York Times* on Feb 25, 2024.
- While Congress isn't supposed to make laws abridging the freedom of speech, the FBI and other Deep State actors regularly induce social

media companies and mainstream media to do it for them.

- They weaponized the Department of Justice to unjustifiably attack political opponents .
- During the COVID-19 pandemic, in violation of the first amendment of the Constitution, they shut down church attendance while allowing liquor stores and strip clubs to do business as usual. Oh wait, that was done by state and local governments, not federal.
- The FBI increasingly instigates crime rather than investigating it.
- U.S. defense spending is 12% of the federal budget. The Pentagon has failed its yearly audit for the last six years. It is a bottomless money pit. The U.S. military has ~750 foreign military bases spread over 80 nations. In 2022, the U.S. spent more on "defense" than the next ten countries combined (in order: China, Russia, India, Saudi Arabia, United Kingdom, Germany, France, South Korea, Japan, Ukraine).

If you're not aware of many of these issues, I invite you to spend less time with mainstream media and more with alternative media. See the Appendix for a few examples of alternative media. In 1976, when the U.S had only three or four national over-the-air TV stations and no Internet, 72% of Americans trusted mass media. A Gallup poll (105) found that in 2023, only 32% of Americans had a "great deal" or a "fair amount" of trust in the mass media. A larger percentage—39%—had "none at all." In view of AI or CGI-generated imaging, it's getting hard to believe anything you don't see with your own eyes, in-person.

Most of the mainstream media (aka legacy media) consumed in the U.S. originates from a handful of companies. From a 2021 essay by Helen Johnson (109):

> In 1983 there were 50 dominant media corporations. Today there are five. These five conglomerates own about 90 percent of the media in the United States, including newspapers, magazines, book publishers, motion picture studios and radio and television stations. As of 2020, the five media giants are **AT&T** (Time Warner, CNN, HBO), **Comcast** (NBC Universal, Telemundo, Universal Pictures), **Disney** (ABC, ESPN, Pixar, Marvel Studios), **News Corp** (Fox News, Wall Street Journal, New York Post) and **ViacomCBS** (CBS, Paramount Pictures).

A similar 2023 report by Adam Levy (120) lists the six dominant media companies as **Comcast**, **Walt Disney**, **AT&T**, **Paramount Global** (formerly ViacomCBS), **Sony**, and **Fox**. I assume it's a little different list due to mergers and acquisitions.

If you're concerned that this concentration makes it easier for outside influencers to control the official narrative, I share your concern. Influencers like oligarchs, plutocrats, CIA, and FBI.

Could politicians be motivated by money, whether legitimate or ill-gotten? They're human and fallible like the rest of us. Consider figures from a 2023 article at Cheapism (106) that compare net worths of recent U.S. presidents before and after office:

- Jimmy Carter: before--$2.3 million, after—$10 million

- Ronald Reagan: before--$10.6 million, after--$15.4 million
- George H.W. Bush: before--$4 million, after--$23 million
- Bill Clinton: before--$1.3 million, after--$241 million
- George W. Bush: before--$20 million, after--$40 million
- Barak Obama: before—41.3 million, after--$70 million
- Donald Trump: before--$3 billion, after--$2.3 billion (not a misprint)

Am I optimistic that the system will change for the better? No, not in the short term. The issues are too complicated for the average citizen to understand and get excited about. More importantly, the well-funded entrenched power players will do everything they can to resist change. Why should they take action to diminish their empires and bank accounts? As a general rule, people don't change until it's more painful to continue as is, rather than to change. That change will probably require a major national financial and/or societal breakdown. Like the Great Depression of 1929-1939. A public short on cash will have to make cuts in healthcare spending so they can pay for food, housing, clothing, and water. They'll also demand a reduction in taxpayer dollars that are funding unnecessary wars, military spending, the surveillance state, and unbridled immigration. When the financial crash or societal breakdown occurs, we'll either return to our roots of lightly-regulated free-market capitalism or go further down the road to authoritarianism or socialism and even worse healthcare. The choice is yours, America.

REFERENCES

1. 6 Reasons Healthcare Is So Expensive in the U.S. https://www.investopedia.com/articles/personal-finance/080615/6-reasons-healthcare-so-expensive-us.asp

2. Mirror, Mirror 2021: Reflecting Poorly (Health Care in the U.S. Compared to Other High-Income Countries) https://www.commonwealthfund.org/publications/fund-reports/2021/aug/mirror-mirror-2021-reflecting-poorly

3. Health Care Spending in the Unites States and Other High-Income Countries. https://jamanetwork.com/journals/jama/article-abstract/2674671

4. Here's the Real Reason Health Care Costs So Much in the U.S. https://www.cnbc.com/2018/03/22/the-real-reason-medical-care-costs-so-much-more-in-the-us.html

5. U.S. Health Care From a Global Perspective, 2019: Higher Spending, Worse Outcomes? https://www.commonwealthfund.org/publications/issue-briefs/2020/jan/us-health-care-global-perspective-2019

6. Measuring Overall Health System Performance for 191 Countries. https://pages.stern.nyu.edu/~wgreene/Statistics/WHO-

COMP-Study-30.pdf

7. 10 Countries With the Best Public Health Systems
https://www.usnews.com/news/best-countries/
slideshows/countries-with-the-most-well-developed-
public-health-care-system?onepage

8. Why Is Healthcare So Expensive?
https://insights.som.yale.edu/insights/why-is-
healthcare-so-expensive

9. West Health – Gallup 2021Healthcare in America
Report.
https://www.gallup.com/analytics/357932/healthcare-
in-america-2021.aspx

10. Getting to the Root of High Prescription Drug Prices.
https://www.commonwealthfund.org/sites/default/
files/documents/
___media_files_publications_fund_report_2017_jul_wax
man_high_drug_prices_drivers_solutions_report.pdf

11. The Unites States Health System Falls Short.
https://interactives.commonwealthfund.org/2017/july/
mirror-mirror/

12. Why prescription drugs cost so much more in
America.
https://www.ft.com/content/e92dbf94-
d9a2-11e9-8f9b-77216ebe1f17

13. Big Pharma's Go-To Defense of Soaring Drug Prices
Doesn't Add Up.
https://www.theatlantic.com/health/archive/2019/03/
drug-prices-high-cost-research-and-
development/585253/

14. Regulatory Overload Report.
https://www.aha.org/guidesreports/2017-11-03-
regulatory-overload-report

15. Politics and Health Care Spending in the United States

https://www.nber.org/papers/w23748
16. How healthcare's Washington lobbying machine gets the job done
https://www.modernhealthcare.com/article/20141004/
MAGAZINE/310049987/how-healthcare-s-washington-lobbying-machine-gets-the-job-done
17. OpenSecrets.org. Sector Profile: Health
https://www.opensecrets.org/federal-lobbying/sectors/summary?id=H
18. Health care industry injects big money in [Vermont] Statehouse lobbying
https://vtdigger.org/2019/01/06/health-care-industry-injects-spending-statehouse-lobbying/
19. Certificate of Need: A Tale of Two States
https://www.birminghammedicalnews.com/news.php?viewStory=568
20. The Cost of Defensive Medicine on Three Hospital Medicine Services
https://www.ncbi.nlm.nih.gov/pmc/articles/PMC4231873/
21. Defensive Medicine Adds $45 Billion to the Cost of Healthcare
https://www.policymed.com/2010/09/defensive-medicine-adds-45-billion-to-the-cost-of-healthcare.html
22. National Council of State Legislatures
https://www.ncsl.org/research/health/state-ins-mandates-and-aca-essential-benefits.aspx
23. Is EMTALA That Bad?
https://journalofethics.ama-assn.org/article/emtala-bad/2010-06
24. American Hospital Association: Uncompensated Hospital Care Cost Fact Sheet (2022)

https://www.aha.org/system/files/media/
file/2020/01/2020-Uncompensated-Care-Fact-Sheet.pdf
25. MSN.com: What Is the Average NFL Salary?
https://www.msn.com/en-us/sports/nfl/what-is-the-
average-nfl-salary/ar-AA1lRSVP
26. Top U.S. "Non-Profit" Hospitals & CEOs Are Racking
Up Huge Profits
https://www.forbes.com/sites/
adamandrzejewski/2019/06/26/top-u-s-non-profit-
hospitals-ceos-are-racking-up-huge-profits/
#49772bed19df
27. Changes in Quality of Care After Hospital Mergers and
Acquisitions
https://www.nejm.org/doi/full/10.1056/
NEJMsa1901383
28. Hospitals are the largest employers in 16 states
https://www.beckershospitalreview.com/rankings-and-
ratings/hospitals-largest-employers-in-16-states.html
29. Health Care's Price Conundrum
https://www.newyorker.com/news/news-desk/health-
cares-cost-conundrum-squared?intcid=mod-latest
30. Why Hospital Monopolies Are What's Wrong With
American Healthcare
https://thefederalist.com/2018/09/28/hospital-
monopolies-whats-wrong-american-health-care/
31. The Provider Monopoly Problem in Healthcare
https://www.antitrustinstitute.org/wp-content/
uploads/2018/08/Havighurst.pdf
32. 2020 Milliman Medical Index
https://www.milliman.com/en/insight/2020-Milliman-
Medical-Index
33. Hospitals & Monopoly
https://www.openmarketsinstitute.org/learn/hospitals-

monopoly
34. The Antitrust Laws
https://www.ftc.gov/tips-advice/competition-guidance/
guide-antitrust-laws/antitrust-laws
35. Guide to Antitrust Laws
https://www.ftc.gov/tips-advice/competition-guidance/
guide-antitrust-laws
36. Price Discrimination: Robinson-Patman Violations
https://www.ftc.gov/tips-advice/competition-guidance/
guide-antitrust-laws/price-discrimination-robinson-
patman
37. The Impact of Primary Care: A Focused Review
https://www.ncbi.nlm.nih.gov/pmc/articles/
PMC3820521/
38. The Effect of Specialist Supply on Populations'
Health: Assessing the Evidence
https://www.healthaffairs.org/doi/10.1377/
hlthaff.W5.97
39. Social Security and Medicare Withholding Rates
https://www.irs.gov/taxtopics/tc751
40. Congressional Research Service
https://fas.org/sgp/crs/misc/IF10830.pdf
41. Excess Administrative Costs Burden the U.S. Health
Care System
https://www.americanprogress.org/issues/healthcare/
reports/2019/04/08/468302/excess-administrative-
costs-burden-u-s-health-care-system/
42. More than a third of U.S. healthcare costs go to
bureaucracy
https://www.reuters.com/article/us-health-costs-
administration/more-than-a-third-of-u-s-healthcare-
costs-go-to-bureaucracy-idUSKBN1Z5261
43. Reducing Administrative Costs in U.S. Health Care

https://www.brookings.edu/wp-content/
uploads/2020/03/Cutler_PP_LO.pdf

44. A dozen facts about the economics of the U.S. health-care system
https://www.brookings.edu/research/a-dozen-facts-about-the-economics-of-the-u-s-health-care-system/

45. Majority of lawmakers in 116th Congress are millionaires
https://www.opensecrets.org/news/2020/04/majority-of-lawmakers-millionaires/

46. AARP, CVS and United Healthcare Keep Prescription Drug Prices Higher for Seniors
https://www.washingtontimes.com/news/2020/feb/11/aarp-united-healthcare-and-cvs-keep-prescription-d/

47. The health care swamp has not been drained
https://www.axios.com/health-care-lobbying-trump-drain-swamp-f2ec6b40-308b-4e10-9fac-a2efae587968.html

48. A Better Way to Fix Lobbying
https://www.brookings.edu/wp-content/uploads/2016/06/06_lobbying_drutman.pdf

49. Hospitals Sue Trump to Keep Negotiated Prices Secret
https://www.nytimes.com/2019/12/04/health/hospitals-trump-prices-transparency.html

50. Safeguarding Pharmaceutical Supply Chains in a Global Economy.
https://www.fda.gov/news-events/congressional-testimony/safeguarding-pharmaceutical-supply-chains-global-economy-10302019

51. Frequently Asked Questions on Patents and Exclusivity
https://www.fda.gov/drugs/development-approval-process-drugs/frequently-asked-questions-patents-and-

exclusivity

52. Comparing the efficiency of health systems across industrialized countries: a panel analysis
https://bmchealthservres.biomedcentral.com/articles/10.1186/s12913-015-1084-9

53. HEDIS and Performance Measurement
https://www.ncqa.org/hedis/

54. HEDIS Measures and Technical Resources
https://www.ncqa.org/hedis/measures/

55. Mandated Health Insurance Benefits Explained
https://www.verywellhealth.com/mandated-health-insurance-benefits-1738931

56. The Effect of Health Insurance Benefit Mandates on Insurance Premiums
https://papers.ssrn.com/sol3/papers.cfm?abstract_id=2107945

57. National Health Expenditure Fact Sheet
https://www.cms.gov/Research-Statistics-Data-and-Systems/Statistics-Trends-and-Reports/NationalHealthExpendData/NHE-Fact-Sheet

58. What's the Average Medical School Debt in 2024?
https://www.forbes.com/advisor/student-loans/average-medical-school-debt/

59. National Health Expenditures 2022 Fact Sheet at Centers for Medicare & Medicaid Services
https://www.cms.gov/data-research/statistics-trends-and-reports/national-health-expenditure-data/nhe-fact-sheet

60. Express Scripts Boosts Cigna As Employers Stick With Larger Insurers
https://www.forbes.com/sites/brucejapsen/2019/08/01/express-scripts-boosts-cigna-as-employers-stick-with-larger-insurer/?

sh=58ca7bc5db1a

61. A dozen facts about the economics of the U.S. healthcare system
https://www.brookings.edu/research/a-dozen-facts-about-the-economics-of-the-u-s-health-care-system/

62. Decline Medicare Part A and Lose Your Social Security Benefits
https://www.verywellhealth.com/do-not-refuse-medicare-when-you-are-on-ssdi-2318713

63. The Principle of Subsidiarity
https://www.acton.org/pub/religion-liberty/volume-6-number-4/principle-subsidiarity

64. PCC, Primary Care Collaborative. Report: Supermajority of U.S. physicians are employed by health systems or corporate entities
https://thepcc.org/2022/04/25/report-supermajority-us-physicians-are-employed-health-systems-or-corporate-entities

65. National Philanthropic Trust: National Giving Statistics
https://www.nptrust.org/philanthropic-resources/charitable-giving-statistics/

66. ICD-10-CM Official Guidelines for Coding and Reporting FY 2020
https://www.cms.gov/Medicare/Coding/ICD10/Downloads/2020-Coding-Guidelines.pdf

67. Intro to CPT Coding
https://www.medicalbillingandcoding.org/intro-to-cpt/

68. Now no doctor's note needed for blood tests in Arizona
https://www.usatoday.com/story/tech/2015/07/02/new-arizona-law-and-fda-approval-gives-theranos-something-to-celebrate/29634373/

69. Excess Medical Care Spending: The Categories, Magnitude, and Opportunity Costs of Wasteful Spending in the United States
https://www.usatoday.com/story/tech/2015/07/02/new-arizona-law-and-fda-approval-gives-theranos-something-to-celebrate/29634373/

70. As of Jan 1, hospitals must publicly list their prices – here's what they won't reveal
https://www.marketwatch.com/story/hospitals-have-to-publicly-list-the-cost-of-care-heres-what-the-numbers-do-and-dont-reveal-for-patients-shopping-around-11609813666

71. Pharmacy Benefit Managers and Their Role in Drug Spending
https://www.commonwealthfund.org/publications/explainer/2019/apr/pharmacy-benefit-managers-and-their-role-drug-spending

72. Pharmacy Benefit Managers
https://www.healthaffairs.org/do/10.1377/hpb20171409.000178/full/

73. Understanding the hidden villain of Big Pharma: pharmacy benefit managers
https://www.newsweek.com/big-pharma-villain-pbm-569980

74. The Growing Problem of Out-of-Pocket Costs and Affordability in Employer-Sponsored Insurance
https://jamanetwork.com/journals/jama/fullarticle/2782041

75. U.S. national health expenditure as percentage of GDP from 1960 to 2020.
https://www.statista.com/statistics/184968/us-health-expenditure-as-percent-of-gdp-since-1960/

76. Exclusive: More Than 70% of Americans Feel Failed by

the Health Care System.
https://time.com/6279937/us-health-care-system-attitudes/

77. Life Expectancy at Birth (OECD Data)
https://data.oecd.org/healthstat/life-expectancy-at-birth.htm

78. The World's Costliest Healthcare
https://www.harvardmagazine.com/2020/04/feature-forum-costliest-health-care

79. Why is Health Care So Expensive in the United States?
https://www.today.com/tmrw/why-healthcare-so-expensive-united-states-t192119

80. Global expenditure on health: Public spending on the rise?
https://iris.who.int/bitstream/handle/10665/350560/9789240041219-eng.pdf#page=11

81. What's behind high U.S health care costs?
https://news.harvard.edu/gazette/story/2018/03/u-s-pays-more-for-health-care-with-worse-population-health-outcomes/

82. Why Are Americans Paying More for Healthcare?
https://www.pgpf.org/blog/2024/01/why-are-americans-paying-more-for-healthcare

83. High U.S. Health Care Spending: Where Is It All Going?
https://www.commonwealthfund.org/publications/issue-briefs/2023/oct/high-us-health-care-spending-where-is-it-all-going

84. Health Care Costs: What's the Problem?
https://www.aamcresearchinstitute.org/our-work/issue-brief/health-care-costs-what-s-problem

85. Why is Healthcare So Expensive? Blame the Lobbyists
https://www.forbes.com/sites/peterubel/2021/04/09/

why-is-healthcare-so-expensive-blame-the-lobbyists/?
sh=7f8f848532e7

86. Hospital and Insurer Price Transparency Rules Now
In Effect But Compliance Is Still Far Away
https://www.healthaffairs.org/content/forefront/
hospital-and-insurer-price-transparency-rules-now-
effect-but-compliance-still-far-away

87. Leading lobbying industries in the U.S.in 2022, by
total lobbying spending.
https://www.statista.com/statistics/257364/top-
lobbying-industries-in-the-us/

88. Scientists Identify the Optimal Number of Daily Steps
for Longevity, and It's Not 10,000
https://www.sciencealert.com/scientists-identify-the-
optimal-number-of-daily-steps-for-longevity-and-its-
not-10000

89. Association of Step Volume and Intensity With All-
Cause Mortality in Older Women
https://jamanetwork.com/journals/
jamainternalmedicine/fullarticle/2734709

90. National Conference of State Legislatures: Certificate
of Need State Laws
https://www.ncsl.org/health/certificate-of-need-state-
laws

91. Statista: Pharmaceutical spending per capita in
selected countries in 2022
https://www.statista.com/statistics/266141/
pharmaceutical-spending-per-capita-in-selected-
countries/

92. CNN: These are the first 10 drugs subject to Medicare
price negotiations
https://www.cnn.com/2023/08/29/politics/medicare-
drug-price-negotiations/index.html

93. Today's Hospitalist. Rising Compensation for Hospitalists
https://www.todayshospitalist.com/rising-compensation-hospitalists/

94. PatientRightsAdvocate.org. Fourth Semi-Annual Hospital Price Transparency Report, February 2023
https://static1.squarespace.com/static/60065b8fc8cd610112ab89a7/t/63dfc34f156b45423beb87b7/1675608912170/PatientRightsAdvocate.org+Feb+2023+Price+Transparency+Compliance+Report.pdf

95. Gallup: Healthcare System
https://news.gallup.com/poll/4708/healthcare-system.aspx

96. Statista: Percentage of respondents worldwide who were satisfied with their country's national health system as of 2019, by country
https://www.statista.com/statistics/1109036/satisfaction-health-system-worldwide-by-country/

97. Ipsos Global Advisor: Global Perceptions of Healthcare
https://www.ipsos.com/sites/default/files/ct/news/documents/2023-07/ipsos-global-perceptions-of-healthcare-2023.pdf

98. The Commonwealth Fund. Country Profiles: International Health Care System Profiles
https://www.commonwealthfund.org/international-health-policy-center/countries

99. Journal of Korean Medical Science: Healthcare Policy Agenda for a Sustainable Healthcare System in Korea: Building Consensus Using the Delphi Method
https://www.ncbi.nlm.nih.gov/pmc/articles/PMC9550634/

100. The Legatum Prosperity Index 2023
https://www.prosperity.com/rankings
101. CDC: Infant Mortality Rate Sees First Rise in Twenty Years
https://blogs.cdc.gov/nchs/2023/11/01/7479/
102. The [Swiss] Federal Council: The majority of the Swiss population is satisfied with healthcare
https://www.admin.ch/gov/en/start/documentation/media-releases.msg-id-99203.html
103. OECD iLibrary: Citizen Satisfaction With Public Services and Institutions
https://www.oecd-ilibrary.org/sites/9c62995d-en/index.html?itemId=/content/component/9c62995d-en
104. OECD: Government at a Glance 2023
https://read.oecd-ilibrary.org/governance/government-at-a-glance-2023_3d5c5d31-en#page1
105. Gallup: Media Confidence in U.S. Matches 2016 Record Low
https://news.gallup.com/poll/512861/media-confidence-matches-2016-record-low.aspx
106. U.S. Presidents' New Worth, Before and After Taking Office
https://blog.cheapism.com/what-presidents-are-worth/
107. JAMA Network: Comparison of Research Spending on New Drug Approvals by the National Institutes of Health Versus the Pharmaceutical Industry, 2010-2019
https://jamanetwork.com/journals/jama-health-forum/fullarticle/2804378
108. Fortune.com: "Turbulence Ahead": Nearly 1 in 4 Americans lack enough money to cover a $400 emergency expense, Fed survey shows
https://fortune.com/2023/05/23/inflation-economy-consumer-finances-americans-cant-cover-emergency-

expense-federal-reserve/

109. The Miscellany News: The unprecedented consolidation of the modern media industry has severe consequences
https://miscellanynews.org/2021/04/29/opinions/the-unprecedented-consolidation-of-the-modern-media-industry-has-severe-consequences/

110. Americans' Views of Government: Decades of Mistrust, Enduring Support for Its Role
https://www.pewresearch.org/politics/2022/06/06/americans-views-of-government-decades-of-distrust-enduring-support-for-its-role/

111. The Commonwealth Fund: International Health Care System Profiles: Singapore
https://www.commonwealthfund.org/international-health-policy-center/countries/singapore

112. Congressional Research Service: U.S. Health Care Coverage and Spending (March 2, 2024 update)
https://crsreports.congress.gov/product/pdf/IF/IF10830

113. Health Affairs, January 2020: Medicare for All: An Analysis of Key Policy Issues
https://crsreports.congress.gov/product/pdf/IF/IF10830

114. Calvin Coolidge Presidential Foundation, March 2020: Debate Brief: Medicare for All
https://coolidgefoundation.org/wp-content/uploads/2020/01/Medicare-For-All-Brief-FINAL.pdf

115. Healthline, August 26, 2020. Medicare for All: What Is It and How Will It Work?
https://www.healthline.com/health/what-medicare-for-all-would-look-like-in-america#1

116. Transparency International: Corruption Perception Index 2023
https://www.transparency.org/en/cpi/2023

117. The Commonwealth Fund. External Reference Pricing: The Drug-Pricing Reform America Needs? https://www.commonwealthfund.org/publications/ issue-briefs/2021/may/external-reference-pricing-drug-pricing-reform-america-needs

118. Contemplations on the Tree of Woe, June 28, 2024: The End of the Deep State? https://treeofwoe.substack.com/p/the-end-of-the-deep-state

119. Politico. Blackburn to Jackson: Can you define "the word woman" https://www.politico.com/news/2022/03/22/ blackburn-jackson-define-the-word-woman-00019543

120. The Motley Fool. The Big 6 Media Companies https://www.fool.com/investing/stock-market/market-sectors/communication/media-stocks/big-6/

APPENDIX

**Alternative Media for Your Consideration
(not for local news, sports, weather)**

By no means do I endorse or agree with everything you see or hear at these sites.

- Tucker Carlson on X (news, opinion, politics, interviews)
- RamzPaul on Rumble (news, cultural commentary, nationalism)
- The Dan Bongino Show on Rumble (politics, news, opinion)
- Michael Farris' podcast "Coffee and a Mike" (interviews)
- "Redacted" with Natali and Clayton Morris on Rumble (news, cultural commentary)
- Jeffrey Prather's "The Prather Point" on Rumble (preparedness, Deep State exposure, communitarianism)
- The Epoch Times (U.S. and international news, lifestyle, health, Falun Gong)
- The Unz Review (cultural commentary, economics, literature, politics, conspiracy)
- Catherine Austin Fitts at Solari.com (for personal finance and investing, banking,

government)
- RT at RT.com (news and commentary from a Russian viewpoint)
- O'Keefe Media Group (citizen journalism, expose wrongdoing)
- Democracy Now! at www.democracynow.org or on YouTube (independent global news)
- Paul Craig Roberts at paulcraigroberts.org (opinion, politics, cultural decay)
- Al Jazeera at aljazeera.com (international news organization based in Qatar)
- Lew Rockwell at LewRockwell.com (news and opinion)
- Alex Jones at Infowars.com (news, opinion, health, politics, economics, conspiracy, vitamins)
- Vox Popoli at voxday.net (philosophy, economics, politics, books, Arktoons, socio-sexual hierarchy, Christianity, classic literature)
- Russell Brand on Rumble.com (news, social commentary, iconoclasm, politics)
- Glenn Greenwald on Rumble.com (mostly politics)
- Stew Peters Network on Rumble.com (social commentary, news)
- Karl Denninger, The Market Ticker at market-ticker.org (finance and politics)
- The Joe Rogan Experience at Spotify.com (long-form interviews with comics, entertainers, politicians, scientists, etc.)
- The Chris Hedges Report at The Real News Network (TheRealNews.com) or YouTube, or ChrisHedges.substack.com (wide-ranging

interviews, essays)

- The Real News Network at TheRealNews.com (journalism "advancing the cause of a more just, equal, and livable planet");
- Elijah Schaffer's "Slightly Offensive" channel at Rumble.com (social commentary, interviews)
- Censored.tv (Comedy and cultural commentary; some free content, much behind paywall)
- Louder With Crowder podcast (Steven Crowder: comedy, news, politics)
- Judging Freedom (Andrew Napolitano) on YouTube (law and politics)
- The Jimmy Dore Show on Rumble.com (comedy, news, politics)
- Timcast IRL (Tim Pool) podcast or YouTube (news, politics, culture)
- Matt Taibbi at www.racket.news and the podcast America This Week (news, opinion, cancel culture, culture war)
- Mish Shedlock at mishtalk.com (economics)
- First Trust Economics Blog (Brian Westbury and Bob Stein) (finance, investing, economics) at https://www.ftportfolios.com/Retail/blogs/ Economics/
- First Trust Market Commentary Blog (Bob Carey) (finance, investing, economics) at https:// www.ftportfolios.com/Retail/blogs/ marketcommentary/
- Futures Edge podcast with Jim Iuorio and Bob Iaccino (investing and finance)
- The Sharyl Attkisson Podcast (independent journalism)
- Larry Johnson, A Son of the New American

Revolution at sonar21.com (foreign affairs, spying, political commentary, war)

ABOUT THE AUTHOR

Steve Parker, M. D.

Dr. Parker has been practicing medicine full-time since 1981. He earned his medical degree at the University of Oklahoma Health Sciences Center in Oklahoma City and did his internal medicine internship and residency in Austin, TX. Dr. Parker left office-based internal medicine in 2001 to be a hospitalist in Arizona.

Dr. Parker has evaluated and treated innumerable patients who had illnesses caused or aggravated by poor diet and inadequate physical activity. His remedial advice would take hours to relay to individual patients. To extend his healing influence beyond the exam room, he shares his recommendations with the world through books and blogs. He wants to keep you out of the clutches of the expensive medical-industrial complex when it's safe to do so.

DR. PARKER'S OTHER BOOKS
The Advanced Mediterranean Diet (2nd edition)
Conquer Diabetes and Prediabetes: The Low-Carb Mediterranean Diet
KMD: Ketogenic Mediterranean Diet
Paleobetic Diet: Defeat Diabetes & Prediabetes With

Paleolithic Eating

Blogs
Advanced Mediterranean Diet (https://advancedmediterranean.com)
Diabetic Mediterranean diet (https://diabeticmediterraneandiet.com)
Paleo Diabetic (https://paleodiabetic.com)

Website
The Advanced Mediterranean Diet (www.advancedmediterraneandiet.com)

www.ingramcontent.com/pod-product-compliance
Lightning Source LLC
Chambersburg PA
CBHW070810220326
41520CB00055B/6841